how to **TIE** a

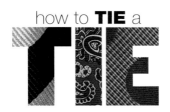

how to **TIE** a

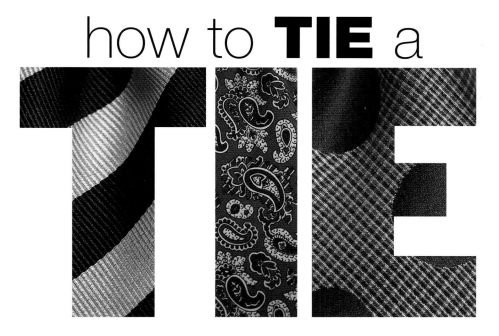

Daniel K. Hall

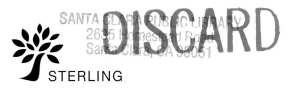

STERLING

New York / London
www.sterlingpublishing.com

Acknowledgments

Thanks to neckties.com and Wildties.com for generously providing ties and accessories. **neckties.** Earth's biggest tie store

Custom ties made exclusively for the J. Paul Getty Museum, Los Angeles, by Winter Design Group.

Tuxedo donation from Fabien Couture.

Photography by Jack Deutsch.

Cover and interior design by Hopkins Baumann

Illustrations by Mario Ferro.

Library of Congress Cataloging-in-Publication Data Available

10 9 8 7 6 5 4 3 2 1

Published by Sterling Publishing Co., Inc.
387 Park Avenue South, New York, NY 10016
© 2008 by Danielle Truscott
Distributed in Canada by Sterling Publishing
c/o Canadian Manda Group, 165 Dufferin Street
Toronto, Ontario, Canada M6K 3H6
Distributed in the United Kingdom by GMC Distribution Services
Castle Place, 166 High Street, Lewes, East Sussex, England BN7 1XU
Distributed in Australia by Capricorn Link (Australia) Pty. Ltd.
P.O. Box 704, Windsor, NSW 2756, Australia

Printed in China
All rights reserved

Sterling ISBN 978-1-4027-2757-3

For information about custom editions, special sales, premium
and corporate purchases, please contact Sterling Special Sales
Department at 800-805-5489 or specialsales@sterlingpublishing.com.

CONTENTS

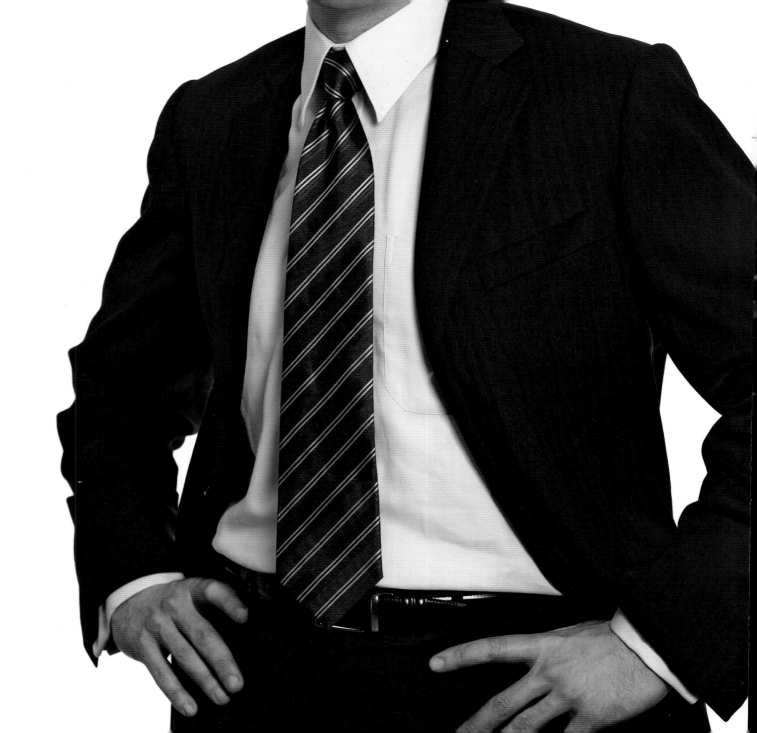

INTRODUCTION

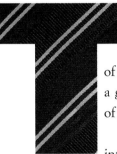RENDS COME AND GO, BUT SOME INCON-
trovertible truths endure.

You're born. With any combination
of luck, savvy, effort, and genes, you're born as
a guy with at least some of the characteristics
of James Bond.

And at some point, you die, having in the
interim (at least proverbially) whiled away
many gainful nights in dangerous company at
a Monte Carlo roulette table, smashed the
twisted leader of an evil empire, bedded a
drop-dead-gorgeous spy or two, and skied the
Matterhorn in a Savile Row suit. You've
probably passed a mirror and noted your
reflection with a wholly due sense of satisfaction at least once.

In which case, you have certainly worn a tie.

Let's, in the interest of likelihood, say
that you've passed a mirror and noted your

reflection with a wholly due sense of satisfaction on several occasions. Mirror hogs aside, odds are high that you were wearing a tie on more than a few of those occasions.

A well-chosen, properly worn tie is one of the incontrovertible truths of men's style. In other words, it's important to get it right.

The average adult male, post–college years, gets dressed (and, if the whole Bond thing works out nicely, undressed) somewhere in the neighborhood of eighteen thousand times. Depending on your profession, calling, and/or sartorial weltanschauung, then, you may be choosing and knotting a veritable boatload of ties. But even if you're not a tie guy, consider the following: job interviews; weddings; funerals; christenings; bar mitzvahs; and the like; and certain cocktail or charity shindigs and soirees.

Also consider:

Both Porky Pig and Pee-wee Herman looked superb in a bow tie.

The string tie did no end of good for Colonel Sanders, who, by mixing and matching it with a lifetime of southern similes and fried chicken, parlayed himself into a household god.

Many a gent sporting a clip-on, poly-blend necktie and short-sleeve button-down has stolen the show at a neighborhood church social.

We rest our case. In other words, our man Bond wouldn't be caught dead in any of these. And with rare exception (such as wearing a bow tie at a black-tie affair) neither should you. Only Truman Capote, Tom Wolfe, and a few other rare flamboyant artists could pull off the tie as everyday wear or party gear.

The fact that you currently hold this little tome in your hands, of course, means that you are aware of the importance of style and that you wish to avoid any of the tie-related style felonies described above. You know what not to do.

But in a post–Casual Friday world where men's style often sadly smacks of the agnostic, even some of the basic dos can be a little elusive. You're not offtrack; you're just not sure how on you are.

What is the standard length and width for straight ties? (Varies some, but a few no-fault tips can keep you feeling confident.) Can a prospective employer or mate standing or sitting five feet from you tell the difference between a cheap tie and a good tie? (You bet.) What's the difference between a cheap tie, a passable tie, and a good tie? (There are a handful of quick tests you can do before buying.) Do you know how to coordinate a tie's weave and width with shirt and suit fabrics and lapels? Can you choose the right knot for the

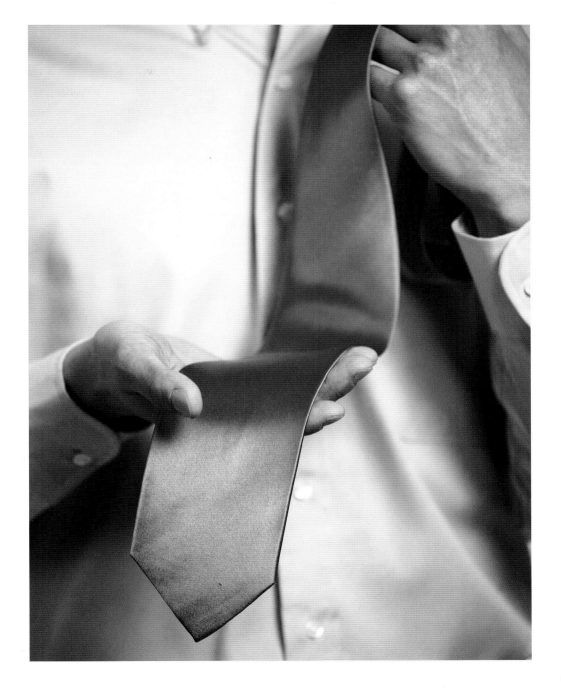

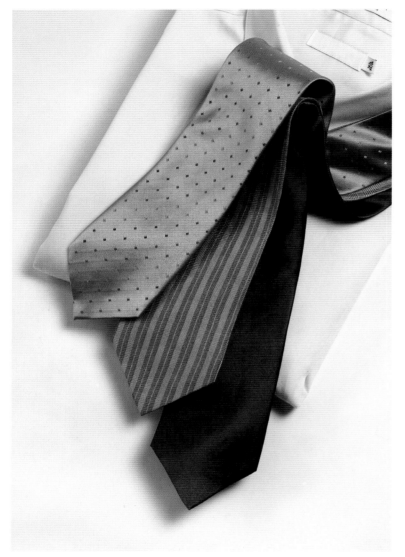

shirt collar? (You will soon.) How much do you know about tie etiquette? For example, is it, under any circumstances, okay to tuck your tie into your shirt? (Never.) And so on.

On the following pages, what you'll find are all the basic rules and regulations of the art of wearing ties (and how to break them, if you choose) along with bits of sartorial encouragement and admonition, as well as some entertaining tie lore and wisdom from style icons on the subject of ties. This is not about fashion consciousness or fuss, just the must-know guidelines, along with a few finer points, for looking good while wearing a tie.

Because, even if you're not gaming in Monte Carlo or skiing the Matterhorn, you want to look good.

Coordinating a tie with a shirt and jacket is largely a matter of personal taste.

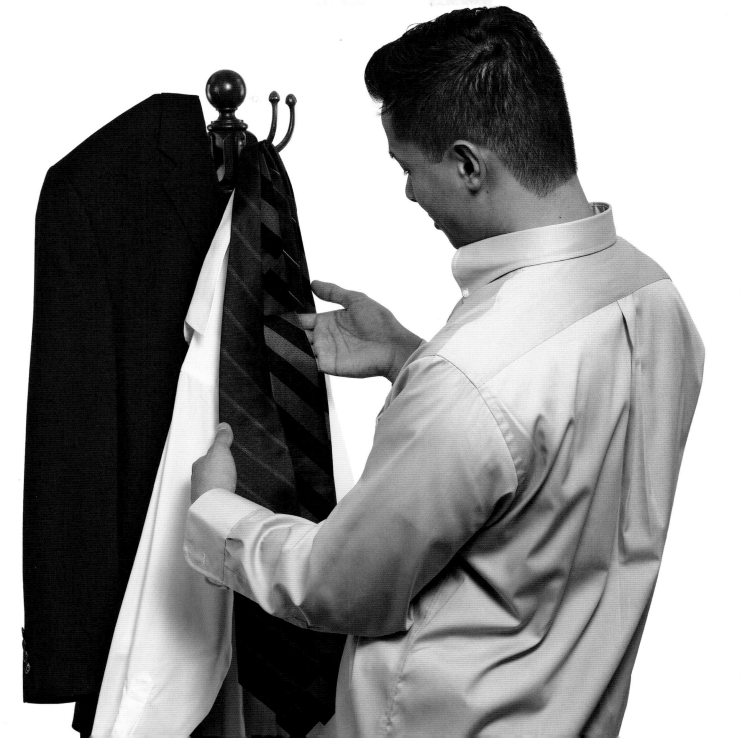

1.
the **HISTORY** of **TIES**

There's never a new fashion but it's old.
GEOFFREY CHAUCER *(1342–1400)*

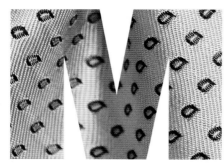

EN HAVE BEEN WEARING TIES FOR A VERY long time. Well, not ties per se—not the kind worn today—but what we might call preludes to the tie. In brief: Various kinds of neckwear have been sported during various eras by various types of men, and from those eras evolved our kind of tie, properly known as the straight tie. While the straight tie itself is a well-designed, orderly thing with clean lines and a no-fuss demeanor, its history is loose and unkempt, with an indistinct point of origin and blurry connections. If history makes you yawn, move on to the next chapters, which will give you all the information you need to look good in a tie in the here and now. But as with all apparel history, the tie has links to economics and sociocultural mores over time and offers up amusing and often provocative food for thought. What follows is a condensed version of the tie's history, with the unbearably tedious bits fished out.

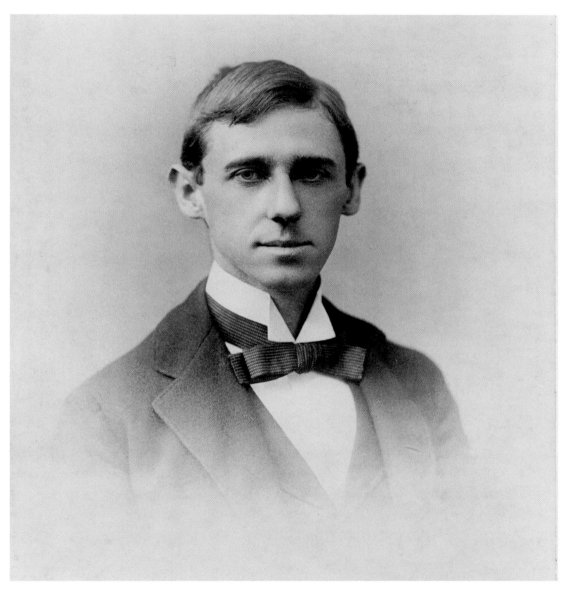

Through its many shapes, forms, and styles, the tie has remained a symbol of male fashion and formality.

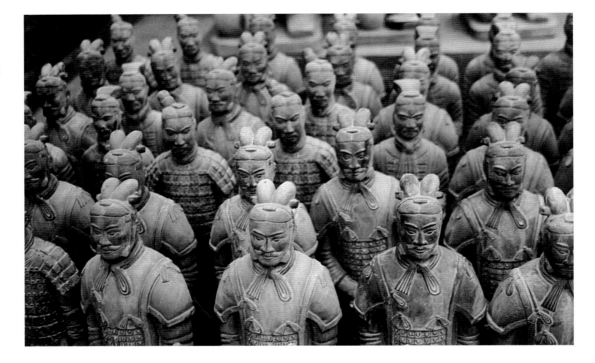

ANTIQUITY:
The Tie's Ties to War

Ties, like many fashion trends and items such as camouflage, parkas, and aviator sunglasses, began as articles of military utility. Hard evidence of gents first wearing ties in combat came to light when, in 1974, archaeologists turned up the buried tomb of the first Chinese emperor, Qin Shih Huangdi (259–210 BC), near X'ian, the ancient capital of China. In it they found an interred phalanx of some 7,500 terra-cotta soldiers, each with a nattily knotted scarf or neckerchief, carved in detail, around their necks. Before this discovery, historians credited the Romans as the "inventors" of men's neck-wear: 2,500 or so sculpted Roman soldiers, many sporting tielike neck scarves, decorate the marble Column of Trajan, a war monument built in 113 AD by the emperor Traianus. (Historians refer to these carved examples of ancient neckwear as focales.) In both cases, purely practical purposes seem to have been the modus operandi behind the neckwear's adoption—it helped keep warriors healthy by protecting their necks from the elements and holding goose bumps at bay. Indeed, it took some centuries for the "tie" to evolve into the ornamental article that we know today, donned by every Tom, Dick, and Harry. Oddly, Chinese cultural artifacts show no trace of neckwear being worn by anyone between its third-century BC appearance and the seventeenth century, when European style dictates began to make inroads into Chinese fashions. And, while the history books show that Romans did don neckwear in the interim, only those most likely to lose their necks along with their ties—that is, soldiers—wore the early forms of ties. Perhaps because of cloth's status as a fairly precious commodity in antiquity, or simply because of a kind of incidental sartorial Puritanism (or not so incidental—with the advent of Christianity, ties disappeared for fifteen centuries), the man on the street went tieless for many centuries. It wasn't until the late 1600s that men began to deck out their necks for fun.

CRAVAT-A-THON:
The (Relative) Fun Begins

The straight tie is descended from the cravat, which itself came of age as a thing of adornment after the Thirty Years' War (1618–1648). France's King Louis XIII recruited a regiment of Croatian mercenaries to assist his troops in waging war against the Hapsburg Empire. True

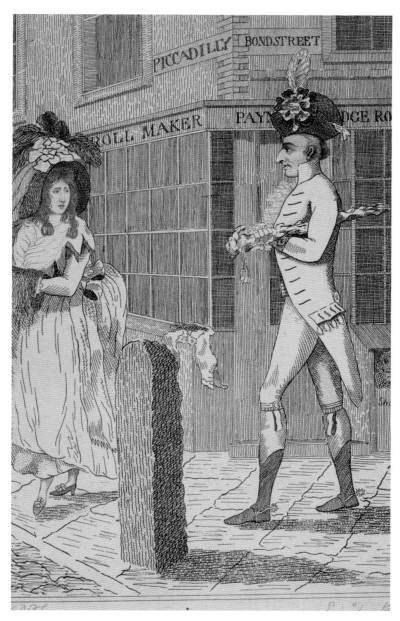

Seventeenth-century style in England and France demanded lacy cravats.

to the tradition generated in antiquity by the Chinese and Roman militaries, the Croats wore knotted scarflike ties, or neckerchiefs—what would eventually be called "cravats"—to keep their necks warm. (Note: The etymology of "cravat" is somewhat murky, with some sources reckoning that the word comes from *Croat*, and some noting the French use of the word *cravate* before the Thirty Years' War. Nowadays cravat is used to describe any type of neckwear, though some wrongly believe it to be strictly interchangeable with "ascot.") The cravat appealed to their French military cohorts, whose own version—a kind of stiffly starched and pressed collar—was cumbersome both to care for and wear. Courtesy of the French soldiers who borrowed the look, the cravat made its way back to Louis's court, where fashionable types incorporated it into the style of the day. From France cravats migrated to England with Charles II, returning from exile in Louis XIV's court. With the Pilgrims, cravats sailed from England to the New World.

The Croats wore knotted scarflike ties, or neckerchiefs—what would eventually be called "cravats"—to keep their necks warm.

The first civilian cravats were made of a length of lace-edged muslin or cambric, or just lace, worn wrapped and knotted around the neck with the ends draped down over the chest. By the end of the seventeenth century, those early cravats were more or less requisite wear for gentlemen on the Continent, in England, and in the American colonies. They were tied in a variety of ways: in bows (enormous, foppish versions of which were later christened "lavalieres," due to their adoption by Louis XIV's mistress the Duchesse Louise Françoise de la Vallière); simple knots, fastened with smaller bits of fabric or ribbon; or in a loosely knotted mode dubbed the "Steinkirk" for its genesis at the 1692 Battle of Steenkerke in Flanders. As legend has it, Louis XIV's troops were roused at dawn by an English regiment's surprise attack; in their haste to rally, they abandoned their usual carefully tied scarf and instead loosely knotted their neckerchiefs, leaving one end hanging down. A more intentional variant of this, with the ends entwined and one popped

Not everyone loved the lavaliere, the enormous bow tie named for the French king Louis XIV's mistress.

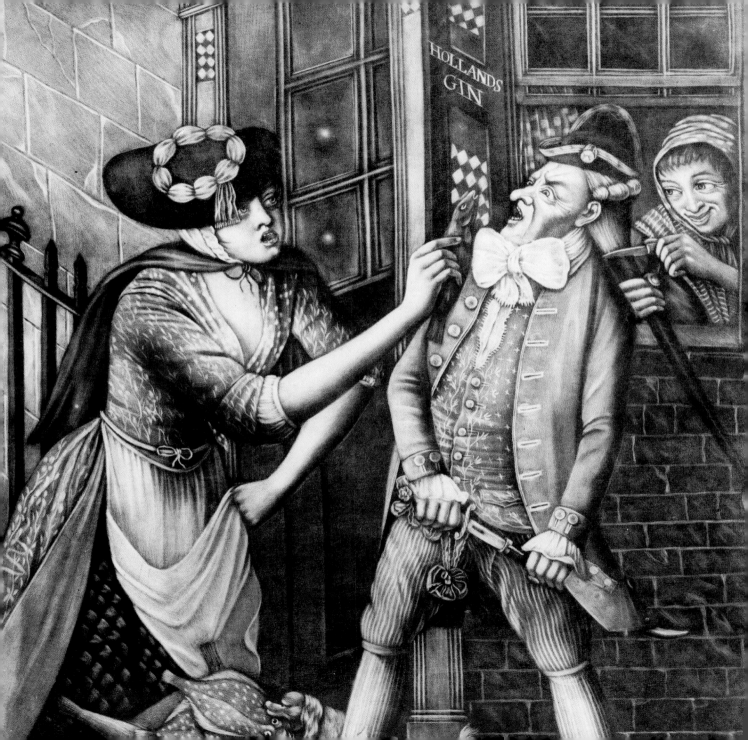

through a jacket's buttonhole, was a style mainstay in England and Europe through the early eighteenth century, and through the century's end in America.

Other forms of neckwear made their mark in the 1700s, most notably the stock—an almost absurdly pared-down version of the cravat, consisting at first of a simple strip of folded white muslin worn plain and fastened behind the neck. Like the ties represented by focales and cravats, the stocks got their start as garb for soldiers (in this case, French and German). Its severe choker style became a fad with youths who saw it as a way to advertise their patriotism, and with its popularity came additions and changes to its make and look. It was often worn with a jabot, a frilly lace front piece, or rigged in a bizarre (but at the time, considered fetching) arrangement with the eighteenth-century equivalent of a ponytail holder, a piece of black ribbon tying back the hair that was wound around and bow-tied over the white stock. (This look was called the "solitaire.") Even with this fancier approach, the stock was a pretty low-key adornment in the wake of the cravat. The cravat, however, was far from having seen its most elaborate incarnation.

NECK-ADENCE:
Macaronis, Incroyables, Beau Brummell, and More

Every era has its rebellions and excesses of fashion, and the latter half of eighteenth-century England saw its rendition in a movement of preposterously dressed society youth whose outlandish aping of Italian fashions earned them the (decidedly politically incorrect) epithet "Macaronis." The Macaronis took their look to theatrical extremes, dousing themselves with colognes and scented oils, embellishing outfits with jewels and baubles and extravagant needlework, wearing enormous white-powdered wigs, and flaunting around their necks impossibly huge, lacy, bow-tied, floppy white cravats. This cry to sartorial libertinism was taken up by the French in the form of a group of men dubbed "Incroyables" (The Unbelievables), the style excesses of which rivaled those of their British predecessors and even outdid them. The Incroyables wore cravats comprising so much fabric that, once tied, the wearer could barely turn his head. (Note: You may be glad to know that America did not host its own band of fashion-debauched peacocks at this time. In fact, the song "Yankee Doodle Dandy," penned by a Brit, famously mocks American moderation: *Yankee Doodle went to town / A-riding on a pony / Stuck a feather in his hat / And called it Macaroni!*

Toward the eighteenth century's finish, the cravat had made a sufficient comeback that it changed form again, seen most often as a largish square of diagonally folded muslin, knot- or bow-tied in relatively modest scale. It was George Bryan "Beau" Brummell (1778–1840), an Englishman whose name has come to be synonymous both with men's style and the sometimes overattention paid to it, who brought the cravat's status to its peak, perhaps paving the way for the tie's eventual importance in daily wear. (Note: The use of the word "dandy" to describe a man with flamboyant or baroque style spars with the word's origin. Dandyism was in fact a reaction against the Macaronis' and Incroyables' over-the-top vogue, meant to focus on a precision of simplicity in dress.) An acknowledged man-about-town and savvy social climber, Brummell was a guy who took his garments seriously, and his attention to matters of dress and infiltration of high society gained him the unofficial but widespread title of supreme umpire of taste. His personal uniform, which predicted what has been the gist of menswear up until today, was a pair of pants tucked into knee-high boots, a shirt and waistcoat and tailcoat, and a perfectly tied white cravat. We're not

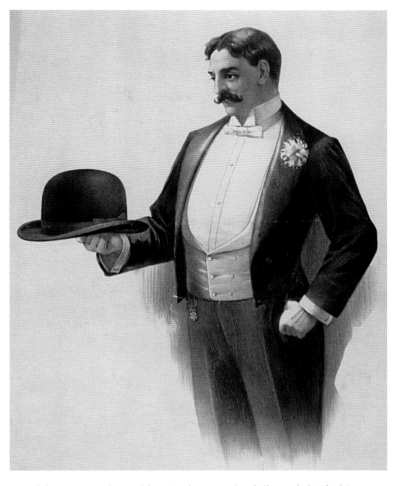

Dandyism was embraced by gentlemen who followed the fashion dictates of the time. Formal evening attire, for instance, required a white tie with a tailcoat.

joking when we say "perfect": Brummell was known to tie dozens of cravats before he was satisfied that one looked good enough to be seen in public. Though presumably few men reached his level of obsession with cravat tying, it did become something of an art, complete with its own social semiotics. French and English how-to publications detailed an increasing number of knots with which the average Joe could tie his cravat; which knot he chose and how well he tied it could signal his social class or inclinations (see below). This explosion of ways to tie a tie may have signaled the widespread adoption of the tie as a guy's real vehicle for sartorial self-expression.

NINETEENTH CENTURY THROUGH TODAY:
Bow Ties, Ascots, and the Tie You Know and Love

If Brummell and his cronies propelled the tie into a way to express themselves, the Victorians, never big supporters of self-expression, were quick to try and nip it in the bud. The hide-it-quick, buttoned-up dictates of late-nineteenth-century Victorian clothing meant that men's jackets buttoned higher at the neck, leaving little room for cravats tied in complex knots. Likewise, the onset of industrialism meant more men who needed practical neckwear that didn't require much time in the morning or much maintenance during the day. The Victorians did and did not have their repressive way: While

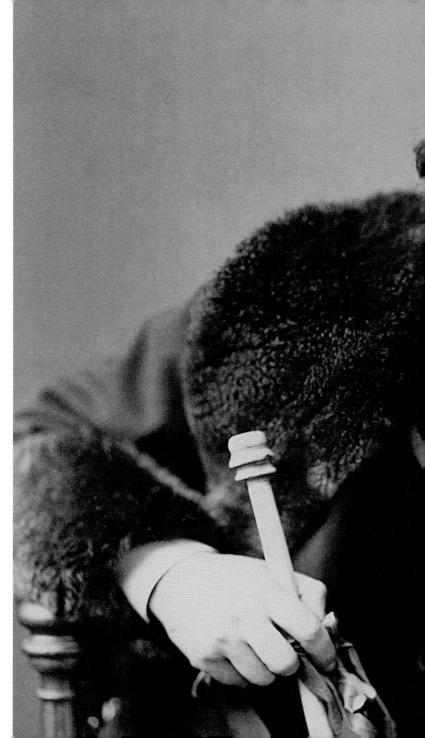

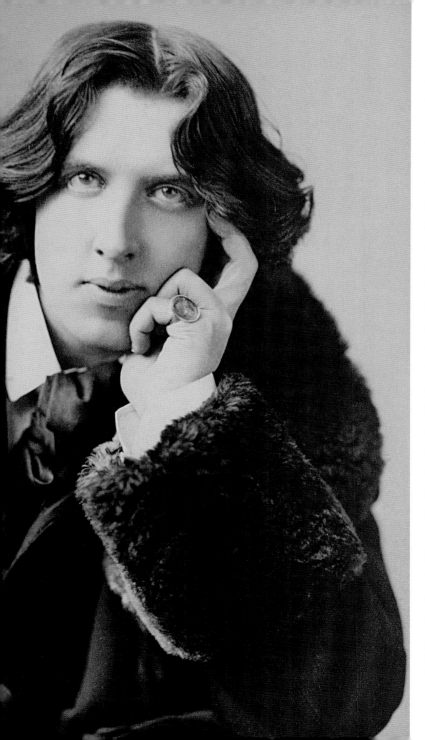

these combined circumstances greatly reduced the number of ways men tied their neckwear, consolation arose in the form of a greater variety of types of neckwear.

The three most popular types are used in varying degrees today. One, the modern bow tie, is basically the Darwinian victor of all types of neckwear tied in bows—the cravat, the lavaliere, and others. As practicality required smaller and smaller ties, two bow-tied versions—the "butterfly" and the "bat's wing"—became standardized (see page 75). The second type, the ascot, more or less derived its shape from a style of cravat tying in which a square piece of cloth was worn with the ends crossed and fastened with a pin; the modern, evolved ascot is more oblong but is tied the same way (see page 84). Both bow ties and ascots found their way into contemporary formal menswear (bow ties for black-tie events being the most obvious instance), and both were put to use (with varying degrees of success) for casual wear, too.

Which brings us to number three: our tie, the tie you know and love, the everyday tie. Of the ties that came during the late nineteenth century and never went, the one that most made its mark was the Four-in-Hand, also

Irish author Oscar Wilde was crazy for stylish fashions. The standard-bearer for the aesthetic movement tied up his look with an ascot.

15

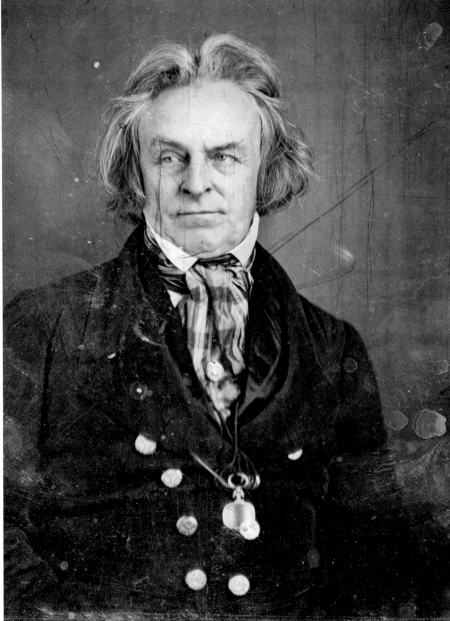

The shift in collar fashions in the early 1800s to softer, turned-down collars appealed to men like southern statesman John C. Calhoun.

known as the long tie, which people adapted and modified down the decades to become what we now properly call the straight tie and, improperly but just as often, simply call a tie. (Note: The first straight tie was initially tied in just one type of knot, and both tie and knot were thus dubbed Four-in-Hand [see page 44].) The Four-in-Hand got its start sometime in the early to mid-1800s, became popular with young British sporty types, and stuck. The first models—often lined with heavy, rough material, just long enough

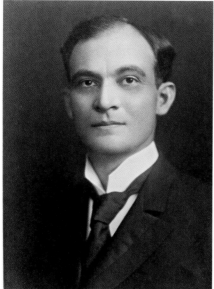

The term "four-in-hand" described the way that carriage drivers knotted their reins, with a four-in-hand knot.

to hide under a waistcoat, and cut straight up and down—were therefore somewhat tricky to knot. Nevertheless their simplicity, along with the shift in collar fashions from stiff and upright to softer and turned down, kept them in widespread use. Invention, as the mother of necessity, produced a wide range of pins, tacks, and clips to prevent slippage from knots and other runaway tendencies.

In other words, the tie in the early twentieth century was holding steady, but it was badly in need of a design rescue. The tie's real hero was a New Yorker named Jesse Langsdorf, who in 1924 patented the design on which all ties made since are based. In a design move as simple as it was genius, Langsdorf constructed ties out of three separate parts (see pages 22–23) and cut them on the diagonal, or bias, producing ties that hung nicely when knotted, whose patterns appeared orderly when the tie was knotted, and whose fabric had enough give to keep its shape better and longer. This process was called Resilient Construction. Since Langsdorf's tie design and construction, many aspects of tie making haven't changed. Through the twentieth century and on into the twenty-first, the decades have proffered radical shifts in tie styles, widths, lengths, colors, and patterns. Beneath the ruckus, the smart, sound architecture of the tie has endured.

2.
how to **BUY** a **TIE**

There is no time, sir, at which ties do not matter.
P. G. WODEHOUSE, *Life with Jeeves*

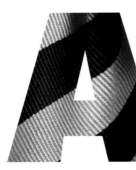

MERICANS BUY UPWARD OF 100 MILLION ties a year and the average American man owns twenty-two, so it's likely you have some in your closet. If your professional life doesn't mandate that you sport a tie on a daily basis, then you've probably donned one for a special occasion or interview. If you haven't yet, you will.

So whether or not you have some already, you need ties. Anyone who has ever entered the tie area of the men's section of a major department store has been daunted by the volume and variety of neckwear from which to select and purchase. You'll be given ties as gifts on various holidays, of course, but we all know what those are bound to look like: chartreuse and red polyester, emblazoned with miniature reindeer. So you'll need ties that are good looking, long

A man's neckwear speaks volumes about his personality and the occasion for which he wears it.

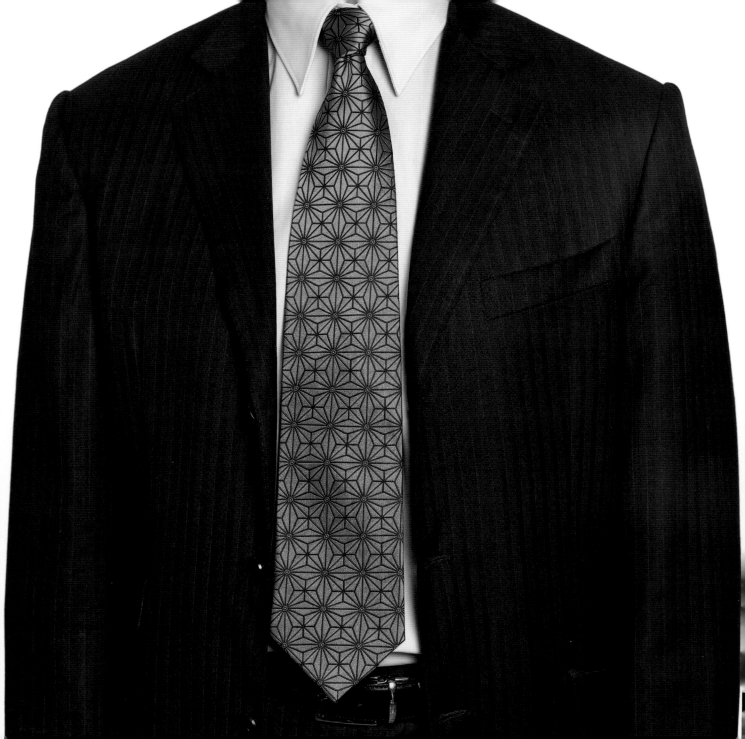

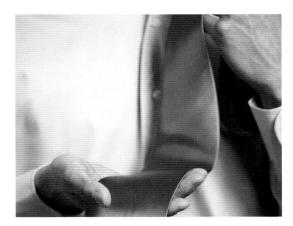

lasting, and versatile, that express your character in a thoughtful, stylish manner. This is something of a tall order and can be tricky to get right. To wit: One of the best things about a tie is that in the relatively monotonous male wardrobe of shirt, pants, and jacket, the tie provides a wide-open opportunity to achieve fashion distinction. However, it also could make you look garish and gauche. Part of what distinguishes the latter from the former is an innate sense of style versus its absence. But the good news is that much of the difference has to do with possessing the right information, such as choosing the right tie to wear with a particular shirt or shirt-and-suit combo (see page 64), but the choice starts with the ties you choose to buy. Buying the right ties can be an easy, inexpensive

The right tie choice will add a necessary and welcome finishing touch to any shirt and suit.
Made exclusively for the J. Paul Getty Museum, Los Angeles, by Winter Design Group.

way to pull together any look, whether casual, professional, or formal.

The following pages tell you how to ensure that the quality, fabric, color, pattern, length, and width of your ties are right so that you look stylish and well put together.

BEHOLD the TIE

Quality is the most important thing to consider when buying a tie, with versatility a close second. At worst, wearing a cheap tie will cost you an interview callback or a second date. At best, you'll be subject to the nagging inconveniences that a cheap tie causes when it doesn't knot or hang well and starts to fray and fade after not much wear. Not surprisingly, cheap ties look and act cheap. Investing in better-quality ties with classic patterns means you'll have better-looking ties that last longer and can be worn with lots of different shirts, jackets, or whole getups. Of course, this doesn't mean you have to start spending lavishly on ties. The best ties will, indeed, cost the most. But there is a wide range of ties by different manufacturers that are well made, handsome, and reasonably priced. By paying attention to the following tips, you can discern which ties are worth their price tags and which are not worth buying at all.

A **TIE'S "HAND"**

As tie savants know, a tie's quality is appreciated by what is called its hand. The hand is the tactile property of the tie, determined mainly by the type and quality of its fabric and the method and quality of its construction and production, which in turn create its weight, texture, volume, and fall (or how it hangs). A fine tie has a "good hand." When you pick it up and lay it across your palm, the feel of it is pleasurable and substantial; as with the taste of a good wine in the mouth, you want the material impression of the tie to linger. It simply feels good, and if you're in doubt, try this: Hold a mass-produced, synthetic tie in your hand, then replace it with a handmade tie of 100 percent silk, or even a mass-produced tie made of silk or a silk blend. The difference in sensation is as keen as that between eating a day-old convenience store doughnut and a croissant minutes out of a Parisian bakery's oven. Become familiar with how different ties' hands feel and you'll soon automatically note the hand of each tie you're considering adding to your stock, and in doing so, increase the quality of your tie collection.

A longer label, stitched farther up the wide end of the tie, often doubles as a bar tack.

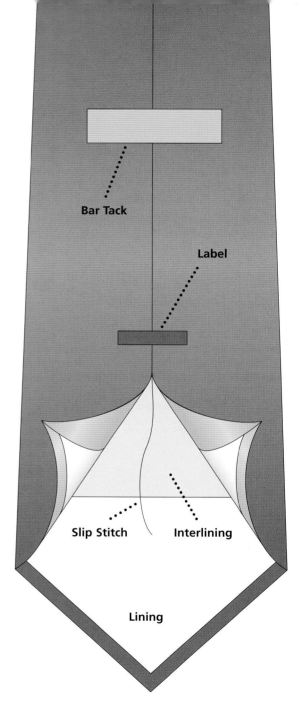

Bar Tack

Label

Slip Stitch

Interlining

Lining

A TIE'S CONSTRUCTION

Like a good martini, a good tie has three main parts. When you're wearing a tie, the part that shows is the external fabric comprising the tie's wide end, narrow end, and often the neckband; this is sewn from two or more smaller pieces of fabric. The parts that don't show consist of a lining and interlining. The lining is made of two pieces of silk or acetate (usually showing the company's logo) sewn onto the back of the external fabric, and an interlining of heavier fabric that is sewn into the external fabric and serves as the tie's skeleton. A 100 percent silk tie lined with silk and interlined with muslin has the best hand.

Along with these structural components, a tie has a bar tack, which often also serves as the manufacturer's label. The bar tack is the small, rectangular piece of fabric sewn into the tie's wide end. It is made of the same material as the external fabric. The bar tack is the bit through which you slide the tie's small end to keep the whole tie in place when you're wearing it. Stitched into the arrow-shaped section at the tie's narrow end, you'll find a little label indicating where the tie was made, what it's made of, and how to clean it.

How the parts of a tie are sewn together is as important as the parts themselves, and you'll learn more about this when we give you a foolproof quality test to run on all your prospective ties to make sure they do the job right (see page 30). However, one bit of stitching is crucial, and warrants mention twice. This is the "slip stitch," a concealed two-to-three-inch (six-to seven-centimeter) stitch located on the backside of one or both of the tie's ends. This tiny stitch is the end of the lengthwise thread used to sew the tie, which forms a little loop and is secured by two stitches that safeguard the seam and keep the lining in place. It gives the tie's overall stitching "play" and thus helps keep the tie elastic and properly shaped, also cutting down on damage to the tie over repeated knotting and removing.

Why's the little thing such a big deal? The slip stitch can only be made by hand, indicating that your tie—even if commercially manufactured—is hand finished. You may have to poke beneath the backside of the tie's external fabric to see it, but make sure to do this. See it and you know you've got a fine tie.

Fabric

Ties can be made of a variety of natural and manmade fabrics, including silk, cotton, wool, leather, rayon and polyester, and both natural and synthetic blends. A tie's fabric is important

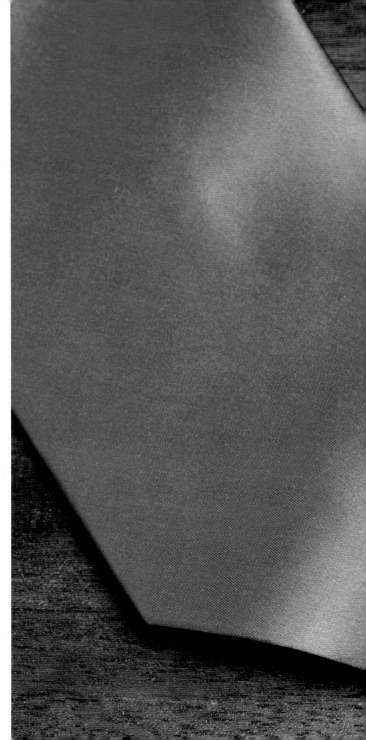

not just for its texture and weight, but also for how it incorporates and maintains color and pattern. While synthetics are widely available and inexpensive, easy to clean, and have a predictable short-term durability, it's hard to ignore that their wash-and-wear convenience is generally partnered with lower-quality designs, hues, and patterns and motifs. Stick with high- or low-end woven or high-end printed silk or other natural fibers, and you'll be in good shape.

Natural Fibers
Silk

One hundred percent silk is incomparably the best material for a tie, though poplin, a silk-and-wool blend, stands just behind it in the quality line. Silk gives a tie a good hand, and this has to do with its texture and weight. The weight of silk, often called "silk weight," is determined by three main factors: the number of threads used to weave it, their thickness, and their weight. (These threads are themselves made up of many tinier, filament-sized threads.) Silk weight is also affected by certain production processes and types of dyes used to give it color. The weave of silk makes it delightful to touch and gives this fabric an elasticity that helps garments keep their shape.

Silk is measured in Japanese-derived units called mommes (MOM-my). One momme is

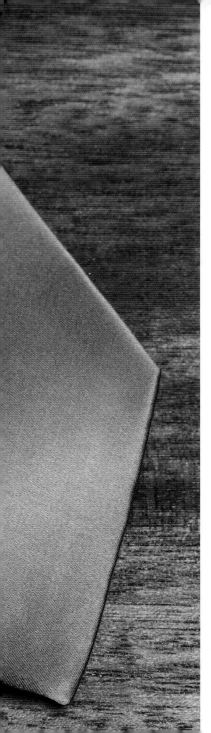

about 3.75 grams per square yard (4.33 grams per square meter). Tie silk is generally between 10 and 45 mommes.

Silk comes in a huge number of stunning colors and can incorporate any pattern or motif. Silk ties are divided into two major categories, woven and printed, each of which hosts a gamut of texture and color characteristics.

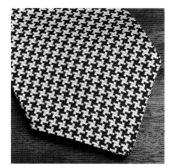

Printed Silk, Houndstooth Pattern

Woven Silk

The man who's a true-blue tie connoisseur wears nothing but woven silk ties. While all silk fabric is woven, the patterns of these ties are woven in different-colored threads into the design of the tie. Because of this, the outlines of motifs are sharp and patterns are well formed; the color or colors used are rich, full, and vivid without appearing jarring or gaudy. Woven silk ties feel best, hang best, and look best. Their weight is ideal, texture satisfying, color vibrant, and pattern perfectly regular.

The textures of woven silk ties vary a great deal and provide a whole realm of exploration. Some handmade, special-order ties use extremely expensive, highly specialized textures such as pleated, flocked, or watered silk. Unusual weaves such as a flecked crepe, basket weave, or their combination can produce beautiful ties of complex craftsmanship. Certain manufacturers specialize in creating

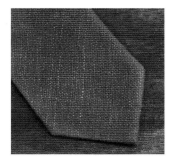

Woven Silk, Unpatterned

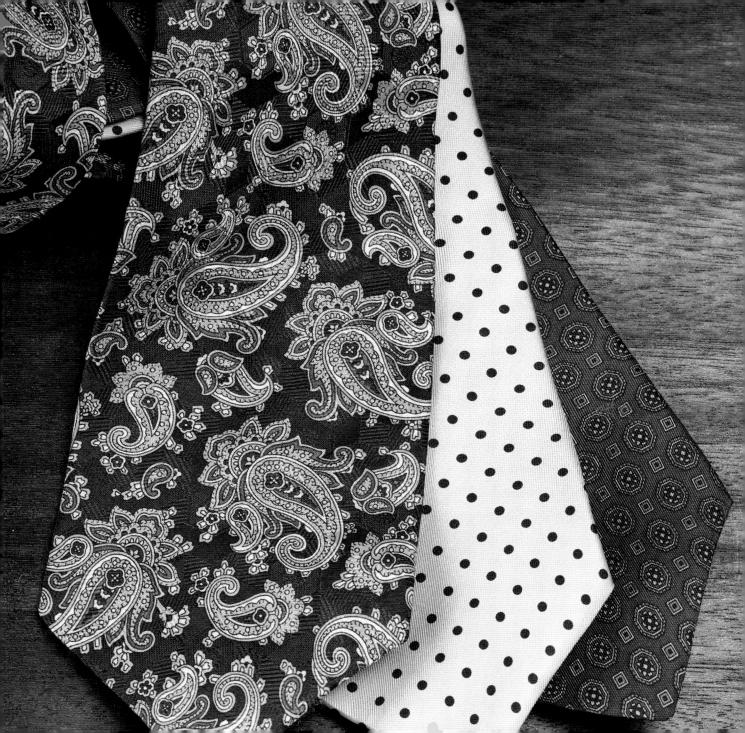

these multiweave objets d'art. Satin weave creates, as you'd expect, a superbly smooth, feather-soft, lustrous cloth. If you own woven silk ties, they are most likely plain weave, the texture used for rep, ottoman, crepe, and faille fabrics.

Printed Silk

Like their fancier woven brothers, printed silk ties offer a wide range of attractive colors and patterns. As a rule, their patterns are not as sophisticated, but they have one big advantage: They are notably less expensive. This combination of quality and affordability makes the printed silk tie the most popular. Unless you're already a bit of a tie aficionado, most of your ties are probably printed silk.

The silk most often used for printed silk ties is of a twill weave, with the tie pattern's motifs applied using a color-by-color screening process. For each color in the pattern, a different screen is used. Portions of the screen are blocked so that only one color can pass through and be printed on the tie; another screen, with other portions blocked, allows the dye of another color to pass through and be printed; and so on. The printed silk for a tie may take anywhere from four to five screens—the most common number—up to twenty-five

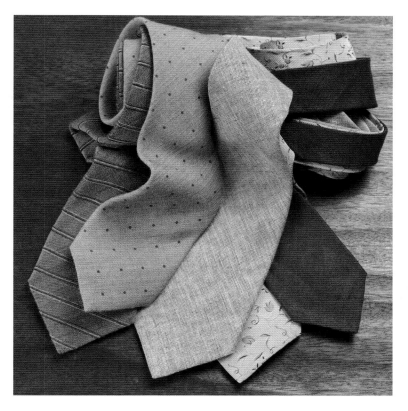

or so. (As the cost of manufacturing these ties is determined by the number of colors and, hence, screens used, printed silk ties with an abundance of hues can be expensive.)

Knitted Silk

Very fashionable in the 1970s but today a bit of an anomaly, the knitted silk tie—with square-finished ends and most often in a solid color—can still make for an interesting look if stylishly paired with shirt and jacket. As an alternative to ties made of woven silk, the silk of this tie is machine-knitted. Its slightly nubby, somewhat slippery texture makes its hand pleasantly idiosyncratic. Take care in taking this one on: Its retro appeal is peculiar, too, and mastering it as part of an overall look takes a man with a clearly defined flair for apparel.

Silk Blends

Poplin. Like pure silks, poplin—a wool-and-silk blend woven with the silk on the surface and wool on the tie's underside—makes a great tie fabric. This special silk-outside, wool-inside weave means that poplin ties are both sumptuous and sturdy, with a wonderful hand (particularly when the wool used is cashmere). Like woven silks, their cost is a bit higher, but their quality of construction and aesthetic, and impressive shelf life, mean they are worth the expense.

Other Blends. Silk can be blended with a number of different natural fibers to produce lightweight fabrics that make great ties for warmer seasons and climes. To this end, silk is sometimes blended with linen or mogadore, a tightly woven mix of silk and cotton. Once in a while, a smidgen of polyester is mixed in a natural-fibers blend to increase its elasticity. (Note: Just a smidgen is the amount of polyester we like in our ties.) Again, these fabrics are not cheap, but economical in the long run.

Special-Effects Silk

Silk can be treated in a number of ways to create extremely luxe fabrics with unusual, sophisticated effects. Pleated silk, washed silk (the silk's surface is washed with sand or pebbles and handsomely roughened), moiré (a highly textured surface achieved by "crushing" the silk) and gum silk (with a more dense, velvety texture) all make stunning ties for more formal occasions.

Other Natural Fibers

Wool

Wool ties, which may be woven or knitted, wear well and can look marvelous. Like the knitted silk tie (see page 27), the knitted wool tie—of a single color and with square ends—had its heyday in the 1960s and 1970s but still makes the occasional wildly successful appearance on the guy with the right attitude and panache. James Bond made the black knitted tie look great with sharp dark suits and crisp white shirts in *From Russia with Love* and other Ian Fleming tales—this, when

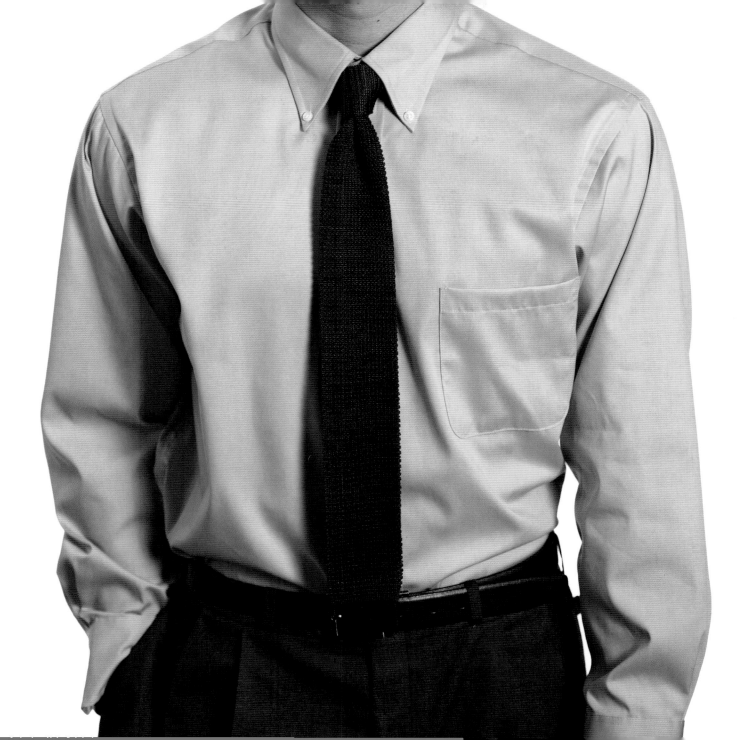

worn well, is considered by some to be an old faithful.

Woven wool ties are made from high-end materials; their heavier weight and cozier textures lend themselves well to winter ensembles. Though harder to find, tweed makes an interesting tie, too—though not for everyday wear. A tweed tie worn with a spruce wool or tweed jacket can make an interesting cold-weather departure from your usual neckwear fare.

Cotton

Cotton ties come in lots of colors and patterns. They are more expensive than synthetics but less expensive than silk. Because cotton is dye-fast, the quality of its color is dazzling, and this aspect makes it quite pleasing as a tie fabric. A cotton tie's hand, however, is less than ideal. It just doesn't feel as good as silk or a silk blend. Like silk, though, it can be worn year-round with casual wear and in summer for dressier occasions.

Leather

A few fashion houses make handsome ties in standard dimensions of leather or suede, and some very stylish guys look good in them. Leather ties skyrocketed in popularity during the fashion-craven late 1970s and early 1980s,

but now they are considered as potentially kitschy as novelty, polyester, and clip-on ties.

Synthetic Fibers

Yes, synthetic ties are inexpensive. Yes, they're easy to care for. Yes, they come in a multitude of designs, patterns, and in all the shades of all the colors of Joseph's fabled coat. Yes, they come in polyester and rayon, and a wealth of blends. If you're a no-fail Jackson Pollock with the marinara sauce and the dry cleaning bills are starting to cut into your mortgage payments, synthethics may be your only option. Otherwise, here's the thing: Polyester ties are about as chic as a polyester jacket.

Quality Test

How do you ensure you're investing in a good tie? Once you're clear on what fabrics work best for ties and how a good tie is put together, it won't be hard to spot which ties are worth their weight in silk. Once upon a time, a man simply had to turn a tie over and check for gold stripes on its lining to know that it was a good purchase. This no longer holds, though there are a few little bits of info and tricks that guarantee you'll spend your money wisely. They are as follows.

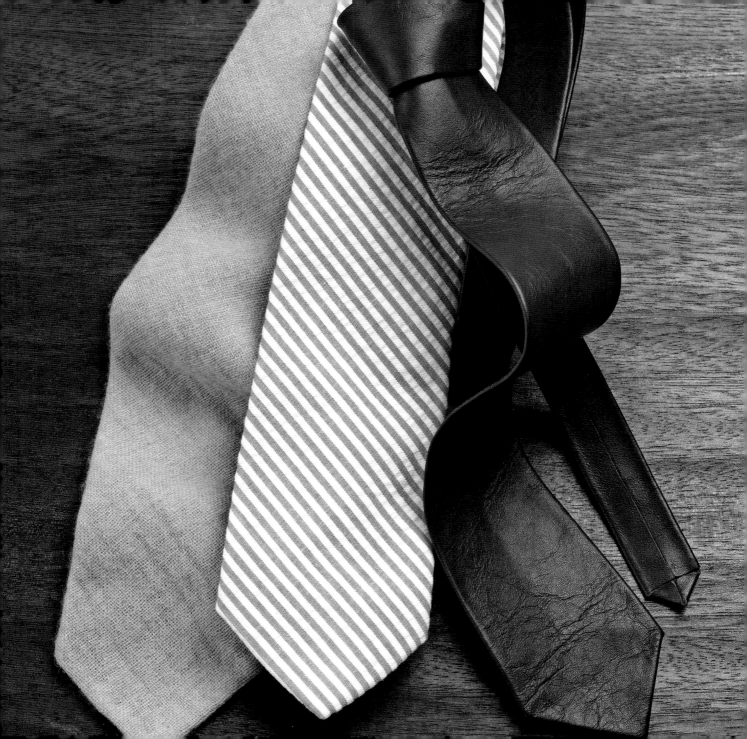

A good tie will have:

▸ a heavier hand (see page 22).

▸ greater fabric elasticity.

▸ a full lining, not just a scrawny strip of it down the back of the tie.

▸ a fine print with clear motifs.

▸ hand-stitching with a slip stitch.

▸ a weave that runs catercorner to its vertical orientation.

To determine that a tie is good:

▸ Hang the tie from its narrow end and make sure that it falls without twisting.

▸ Let the tie hang over your forearm and make sure that its narrow end is centered against the wide end.

▸ Check its elasticity by giving it a yank at both ends; it should bounce back to its original shape right away.

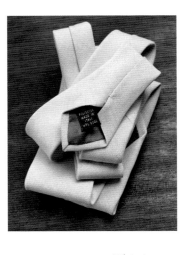

Make sure the tie's lining is securely stitched to the external fabric (the part of the tie that shows when you're wearing it) and that it doesn't shift or slide over when you pull it. Look at the seams that secure the lining to the tie and make sure that they are strong and that they extend far enough upward to conceal the interlining. Under the back seam of the tie's external fabric, be sure there's a slip stitch (see page 23) there. This ensures that the tie's been hand-finished, will maintain its elasticity and shape, and will retain its shape after umpteen knottings and loosenings.

COLOR and PATTERN

Good ties, whether made of silk or other fabric, come in many colors and many patterns.

Understanding how ties of different fabrics are produced gives you a healthy grasp on how the make and cloth of a tie influence the quality of its color and pattern. In short, the better the tie, the richer and more lush the color and the more crisp and/or intricate the pattern. These are not minor details; they are critical ones.

This is not to say that you must develop any Matisse-like knack for palette and composition, just a sense of what colors, shades of colors, and motifs suit your wardrobe, facial complexion and shape, and personality. When it comes to color and pattern, the real challenge is that Sphinx-worthy riddle: Which tie to wear with which shirt and jacket? We'll get to that. In the

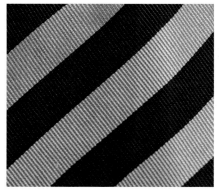

Regular Stripes

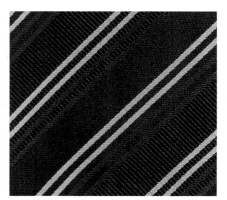

Ribbon

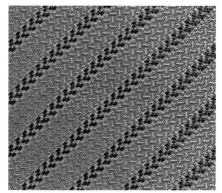

Titan

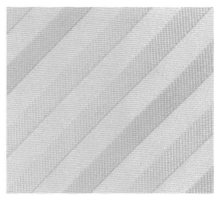

Shadow

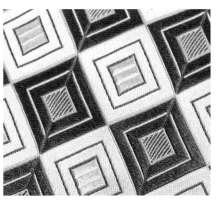

Heraldic

Bandolier

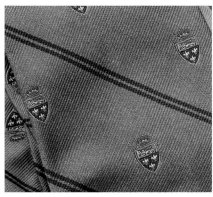

Club

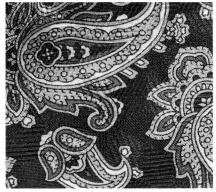

Geometric

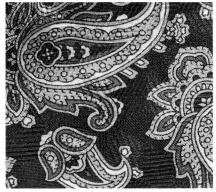

Paisley

Stripes are one of the most basic of tie patterns and also among the most fashionable. Whether uniform and diagonal or tricolored and variable in width, a striped tie is a dependable choice for all occasions.

Paisley is a pattern that conjures up images of book-lined studies and tweed blazers: wisdom, refinement, and venerability. It's an excellent choice for those who'd like to add some intelligence to their lives. Due to its associations with scholarly eccentricity, however, it's best to proceed with caution.

Animal and flower prints represent the greatest challenge in tie fashion: On the one hand, they are powerful statements of personality, the most fully formed and figurative statements one could make on a tie. On the other hand, they're also the lowest circle in the tie commedia: One sparkly eyed–puppy misstep and you may have committed an unforgivable tie fashion sin.

▼ ▲ ▼ ▲

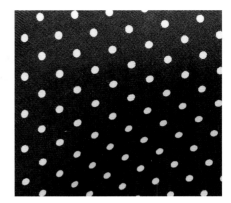

Dotted

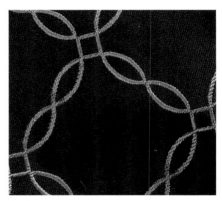

Custom

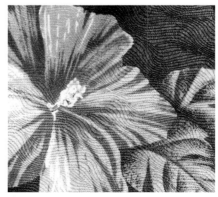

Floral

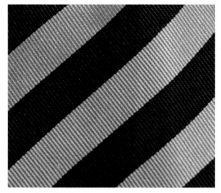

Regular Stripes

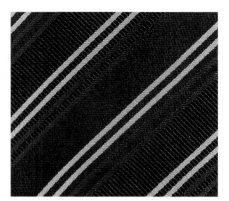

Ribbon

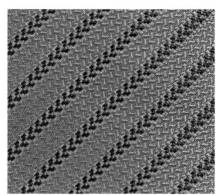

Titan

Shadow

Heraldic

Bandolier

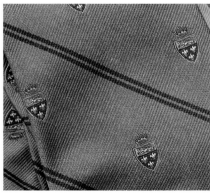

Club

Geometric

Paisley

35

Stripes are one of the most basic of tie patterns and also among the most fashionable. Whether uniform and diagonal or tricolored and variable in width, a striped tie is a dependable choice for all occasions.

Paisley is a pattern that conjures up images of book-lined studies and tweed blazers: wisdom, refinement, and venerability. It's an excellent choice for those who'd like to add some intelligence to their lives. Due to its associations with scholarly eccentricity, however, it's best to proceed with caution.

Animal and flower prints represent the greatest challenge in tie fashion: On the one hand, they are powerful statements of personality, the most fully formed and figurative statements one could make on a tie. On the other hand, they're also the lowest circle in the tie commedia: One sparkly eyed–puppy misstep and you may have committed an unforgivable tie fashion sin.

▼▲▼▲

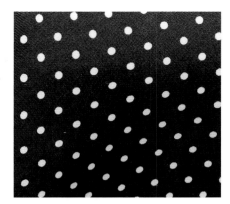

Dotted

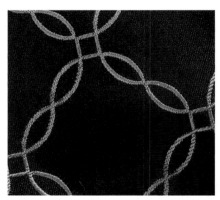

Custom

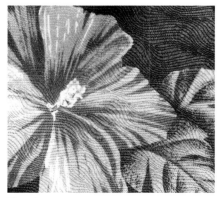

Floral

Other Common Patterns

Though the list of potential patterns is vast, there are a few other themes that make markedly regular tie appearances.

Art Ties. This category claims tie patterns inspired by famous works of art, and individual or series of ties created by famous artists. The former are found more commonly, often bestowed upon the wearer as a gift from a museum catalog. Impressionism tends to figure prominently as a style, though you can find ties with images of anything from Italian Renaissance art to cubism, pop art, and beyond. In general, it's best to avoid these, though well-made versions with subtler motifs or images can work once in a long while.

Ties have long had a link to art and artists. The Italian futurists dabbled in creating various types of eccentric, colorful ties. Dalí produced ties for sale in the 1940s; Picasso famously painted a tie blue and presumably made a mint selling it to the highest bidder. You may find an artist-made tie that's terrific—they do exist. Just be aware of that not-so-fine line between terrific and tacky.

Sports Ties. The English have long been big on ties with symbols associated with hunting, various equestrian pursuits, the green and tee, fishing, and other traditionally upper-class leisure activities that take place in the Great Outdoors. Some American anglophiles have adopted this style, though the coveted *Brideshead Revisited* import is somewhat lost in transatlantic versions. Fine ties with subtle sports-related all-over patterns—miniature tennis rackets, polo players, and so on—are perfectly fine to wear in casual contexts that allow for their boyish effect. But showing support for your favorite team via the tie—boyish or not—should be avoided at all costs. This means no ties with large basketballs printed on them, nor the name of your favorite team, nor your favorite player's name spelled out in bold, team-spirit calligraphy. You'll thank us in the future.

Novelty Theme Ties. We speak here of the Donald Duck tie; of the thin black tie with white piano keys running down its length; of the tie that offers up Santa, apple cheeked and achortle, waving as he descends, present-laden, into the chimney; and their neckwear compadres. There's no upgrading the wisdom put forth on this subject by writers Scott Omelianuk and Ted Allen, who addressed it best in their book *Esquire's Things a Man*

Should Know About Style: "Wit or humor is never to be expressed through a tie." Generally speaking, the same thing goes for patriotism and religion, and allegiance to television shows, hot rods, or rock bands. (See also page 88.)

DIMENSIONS

Buying good quality will largely ensure that your ties have the right dimensions. But like the rise and fall of women's hemlines and the widths of shirt and jacket lapels, ties are worn wider or skinnier, longer or shorter, depending on the decade. There are certain dimensions that endure and allow the tie to knot, hang, and look best.

A tie should be:

▸ approximately 3.5 inches wide. If worn with a suit, the tie's width should approximate the lapels of the suit.
▸ 55 to 56 inches long. When worn, the tie's point should cover the belt buckle but never fall below the belt buckle.

FANCIER TIES

Ties may be made almost wholly by machine, by machine with hand finishing, or completely by hand. Machine-manufactured ties with hand finishing account for the greatest percentage of higher-quality ties on the market and are probably what make up most of your tie wardrobe. Manufacturers make many of each design, and they are thus affordable, while still attractive and well made. If you want a tie that's truly a work of craftsmanship, or one of a kind, here are your other options.

Handmade Ties

Handmade ties are the work of real craftsmen, tie specialists who ply their trade in small studios producing very limited editions of tie designs. Their work is superb, with careful attention and care paid to all stages of the tie's construction, and the ties they create are top of the line. As with all things of great quality, they can cost a bundle. But if they're well cared for, they'll last a lifetime and likely still be in good enough shape to hand down to a son or nephew eventually. A word to the wise: The "handmade" label does not necessarily mean handmade. Many foreign companies ship boatloads of manufactured ties to the United States and have the "handmade" label sewn on by hand (as if this process itself warranted the label). In other words, know your vendor.

Custom-Made Ties

You'll find custom ties few and far between these days, though some boutique haberdashers and fashion houses, largely European, still offer custom service. A man may decide to have a tie custom made because he has particular, personal requirements, likes, or dislikes with regard to the designs of standard ties. Most often, though, the request for a custom-made tie comes because he's taller, shorter, or broader than average. But some more esoteric tie knots and certain shirt collars require that a tie be longer or wider, too.

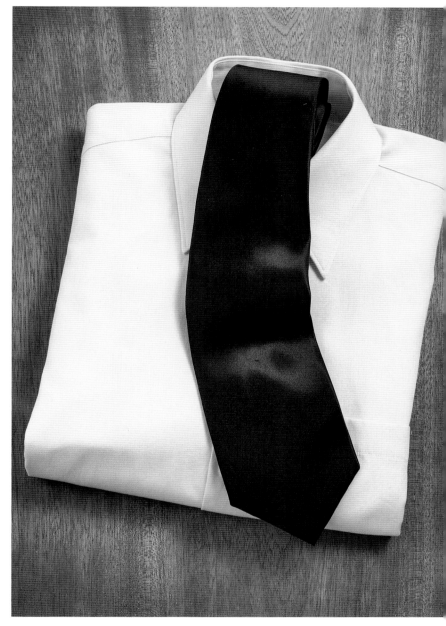

3.
how to **KNOT** a **TIE**

The art of the tying of ties is for the man of the world what the art of giving dinners is for the statesman.

ÉMILE MARC HILAIRE,
ALIAS MARCO DE ST. HILAIRE,
French writer, 1793–1887

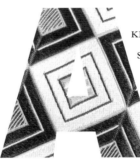

A KNOT, LIKE A MAN WEARING A TIE WITH self-assurance, has gravitas. Knots mean business: For centuries in cultural ritual, myth, language, and literature, knots have symbolized creation, union, strength, fecundity, mystery, dilemma, solution—all the serious subjects of what Shakespeare called "this mortal coil" of life and death. A guy in a tie means business, too—even if that business has nothing to do with commerce and has simply to do with looking his best. The point is that if you're going to wear a tie, you need to be able to knot the tie well. Of course, ready-tied and clip-on straight ties do exist, but so do rainbow suspenders and other less than elegant garments.

Approximately four thousand types of knots exist, according to *The Ashley Book of Knots.*

Having the skills and know-how to create the appropriate knot can make or break a tie wearer.

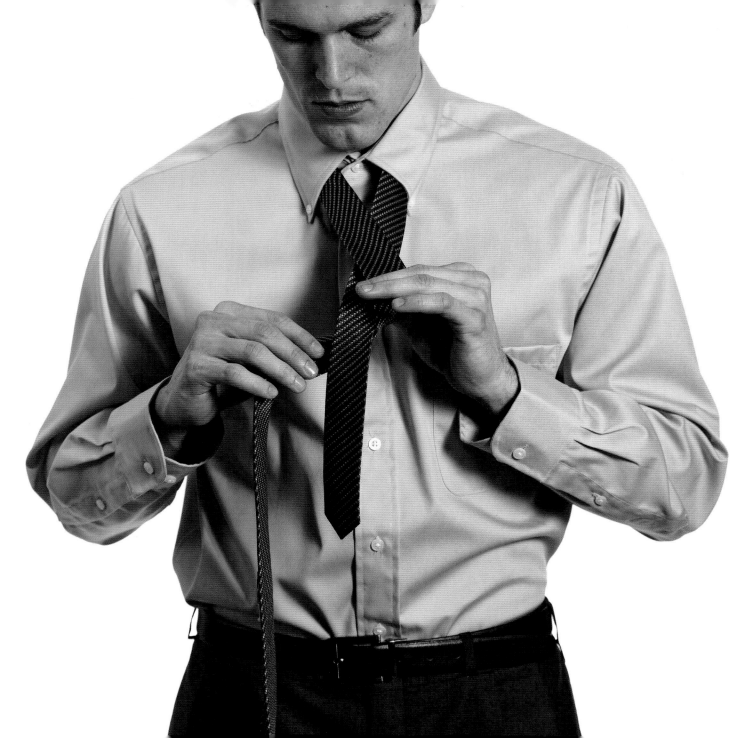

Close to a hundred can be used to tie a tie, according to tie-knot specialists Thomas Fink and Yong Mao (*The 85 Ways to Tie a Tie: The Science and Aesthetics of Tie Knots*, 4th Estate/HarperCollins, 2001), two Cambridge theoretical physicists who derived eighty-five knots that range from standard ones composed of three simple moves to trickier ones requiring eight or nine passes, loops, and tucks. If the idea of fiddling with eighty-five knots satisfies your intellectual curiosity or style bent, you're golden. But if you just want to look put together in your daily life, you need to know how to tie only a few of those, and you're about to find out everything you need to know about tying them. These are the Four-in-Hand, Windsor, Half-Windsor, and Pratt (sometimes also known as the Shelby).

Learning to knot a tie is in the same skill-acquisition camp as riding a bicycle or driving a car. It comes naturally but requires practice for perfection. Although tying a tie doesn't take long to learn, once you've got the basics down you never forget how to do it. The more you do it, the better you get. This is not to say people haven't been frustrated by trying to tie a tie. The most striking and comical example is that of the legendary nineteenth-century dandy George Bryan "Beau" Brummell, who was rumored to routinely stand amid a veritable mountain of discarded, imperfectly tied cravats, continuing to knot tie after tie until, relentlessly focused on sartorial transcendence, he got it just right.

Even in Brummell's day, there were a lot of knots from which to pick. A series of how-to treatises and books on tie-tying came out in England and France in the early 1800s, from *Neckclothitania; or Tietania*, which in 1818 offered up a dozen trendy styles; to 1827's *L'art de se Mettre sa Cravate*, proffering thirty-two "knots" for cravats; to *L'art de la Toilette* in 1830, which illustrated a whopping seventy-two ways to tie a cravat. The French, not content to simply outdo the English in this style matter, had to one-up even themselves. The Brits, in the form of Fink and Mao, upped the ante again.

On the next few pages, you'll find step-by-step instructions for the most commonly used tie knots. You may just like the looks of one, or find it suits you and your wardrobe better, and stick with that. That's okay. While some European men still use lots of different kinds of knots, most American and British men stick with one or two. On the other hand, it's good to know a few other knots to change it up some for different shirt collars, types of ties, and occasions. For that reason, we've added three extra good-looking, versatile, slightly more esoteric knots: the Prince Albert, Oriental, Cavendish, and Nicky.

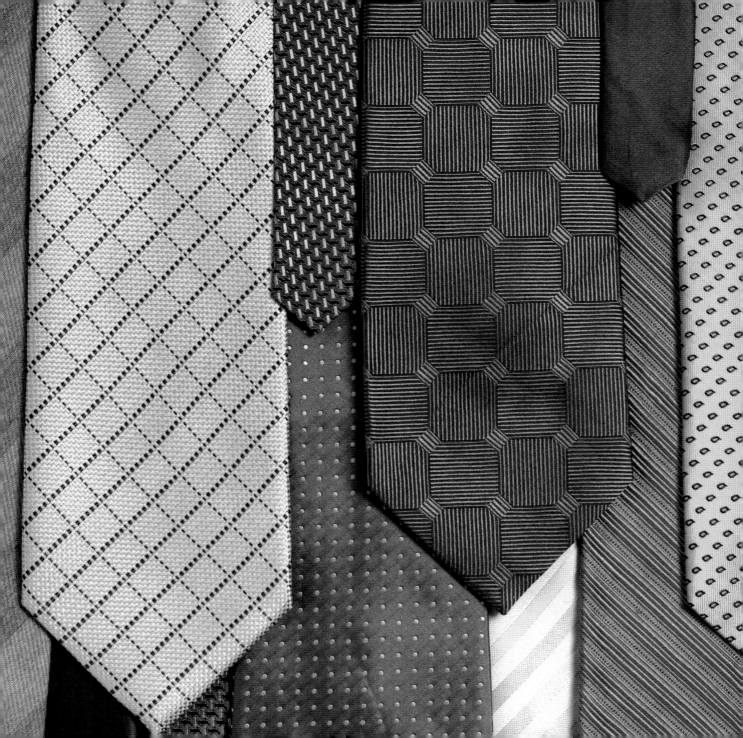

The **BASICS:**
The **FOUR-IN-HAND**

If you know how to tie a tie already, and know just one knot, this is most likely it. The Four-in-Hand was the first tie knot invented and arguably still the easiest to tie among those commonly used. The knot's origins and etymology are shrouded in confusion, and there is no exact date as to when it first made its way around a gentleman's neck. It likely made its debut around the middle of the nineteenth century in England, right around the time when the prototype of the straight tie made its appearance, too—both tie and knot were called Four-in-Hand.

Why this name? Tie lore tells it a few different ways. At the eighteenth century's close, a four-horse carriage driven by a single man was referred to as a Four-in-Hand. It is possible that the carriage drivers tied the reins in what came to be called a Four-in-Hand knot and that they wore neckties knotted in that fashion. During that same period, a London gentleman's club also claimed the name "The Four-in-Hand," where members may well have tied their neckware in the Four-in-Hand fashion, with the knot's name a natural outcome.

Whatever its true genesis, the Four-in-Hand knot stuck, in large part due to its tidy look and easy-to-tie appeal. With the Industrial Revolution and the growth of the workforce, more men had to wear ties to the office every day and didn't have time to fuss with fancier neckwear. Around this time, upper-class men were also looking for something less complicated to wear for leisure pursuits such as sports and travel. It quickly became the knot for the average guy. Until the 1930s, when the Windsor knot was introduced, the Four-in-Hand was pretty

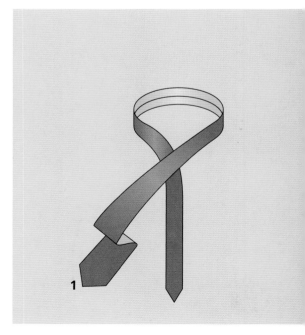

much the only tie knot around, and it remains today a standard of American and British menswear. Because it doesn't require loads of moves and therefore doesn't steal a tie's ultimate length, it's a great bet for taller men, and its slender, somewhat triangular shape complements and downplays a rounder face in ways that some of the bulkier knots do not. It works best with heavier-weight ties and is best combined with small-spread or tab collars (see page 64).

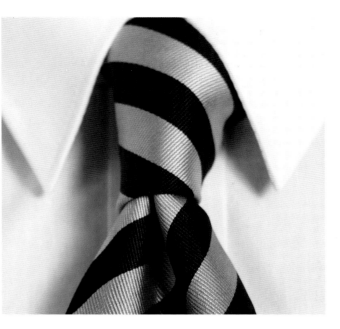

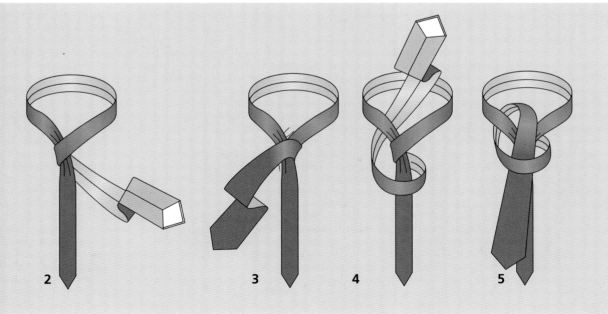

2   **3**   **4**   **5**

The **WINDSOR**

England's duke of Windsor is erroneously associated with this knot even though he never wore his tie knotted that way. On the contrary, the duke used a Four-in-Hand knot with a very thick tie that gave it the volume of a Windsor knot, for which it was mistaken. (The knot kept the name even after photographer Lord Lichfield snapped the duke in a series of how-to shots demonstrating that he didn't use the Windsor knot.) Yet, albeit in a somewhat oblique manner, the duke of Windsor was responsible for the Windsor knot's popularity. He was coronated Edward VIII in 1936, and his abdication from the throne to marry the twice-divorced American Wallis Simpson catapulted him into the media spotlight. Style watchers noted his dashing use of a larger, bulkier tie knot and hopped on the bandwagon, using the Windsor knot they believed the duke preferred.

The Windsor, referred to sometimes as a Full Windsor, is the largest of the more common knots used today. It's also an easy knot to tie, but you'll want a longer tie to achieve the knot and still have your tie hang well. If you find that whenever you wear your tie, it still hangs a little too low, you may want to give this

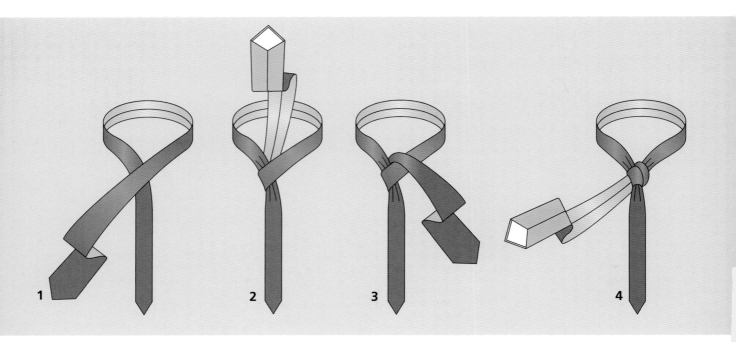

1

2

3

4

knot a try. You need a little room to accommodate its volume, so wear it with a widespread collar.

The Windsor isn't for absolutely everyone. Some consider it a look of slightly bygone days. James Bond "mistrusted anyone who tied his tie with a Windsor knot. It showed too much vanity. It was often the mark of a cad," wrote Ian Fleming in *From Russia with Love.* But at the end of the day, the Windsor is a fine knot hailing from a fine tradition. It bespeaks a tad more attention paid to style than the Four-in-Hand or Half-Windsor, but it is hardly the signature of conceit.

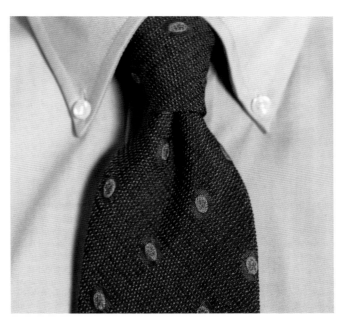

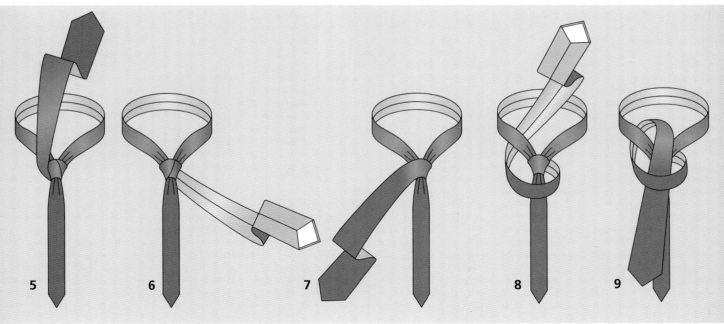

5   6   7   8   9

The **HALF-WINDSOR**

Believe it or not, the Half-Windsor is not actually a variation of the Windsor. Nor is it 50 percent as big as a Windsor but more like 75 percent the Full Windsor's size.

Nevertheless, the Half-Windsor is a knot worth knowing. In regular use since the 1950s, it makes a great everyday knot: Medium-sized and evenly proportioned, it looks good with a lot of different face shapes, suits a variety of tastes, and works with almost any type of shirt collar. Use it to knot a lightweight tie and you'll get a modest look; knot a heavier tie with it and you'll get a little more volume. Some men who wear a slightly wider tie add a final touch to their Half-Windsor knots by giving the fabric immediately below the finished knot a gentle press with a finger, creating a tiny indentation or "dimple."

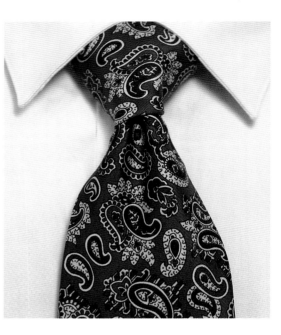

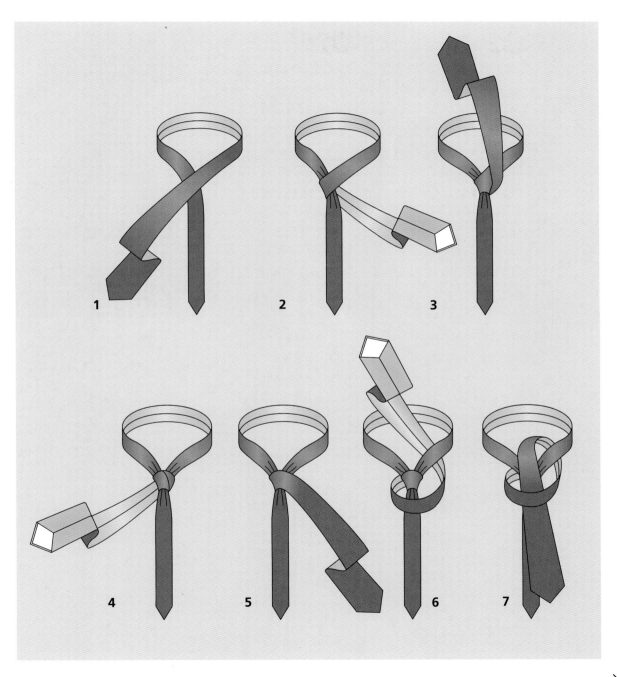

1   2   3

4   5   6   7

The **PRATT** or **SHELBY**

The Pratt was introduced to the world at large via the *New York Times* and *New York Daily Telegraph* in 1989. Its inventor, an unsuspecting U.S. Chamber of Commerce worker named Jerry Pratt, had been tying his tie this way for thirty-odd years when, one day, Minnesota anchorman Don Shelby tried it on for size and received a lot of attention. The less visible Pratt was overlooked as the media dubbed the newly "discovered" knot the Shelby. In fact, it had been worn in the United States as early as World War II. (At that time it was referred to as a Reverse Half-Windsor, despite the fact that its configuration is in no way the opposite of the Half-Windsor, which as you now know, is itself not half of a Windsor.) It's a versatile knot that goes anywhere, anytime, with any man.

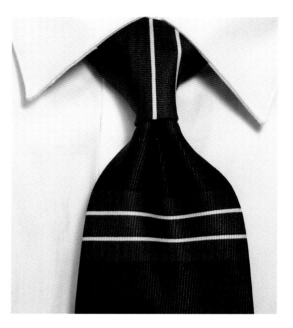

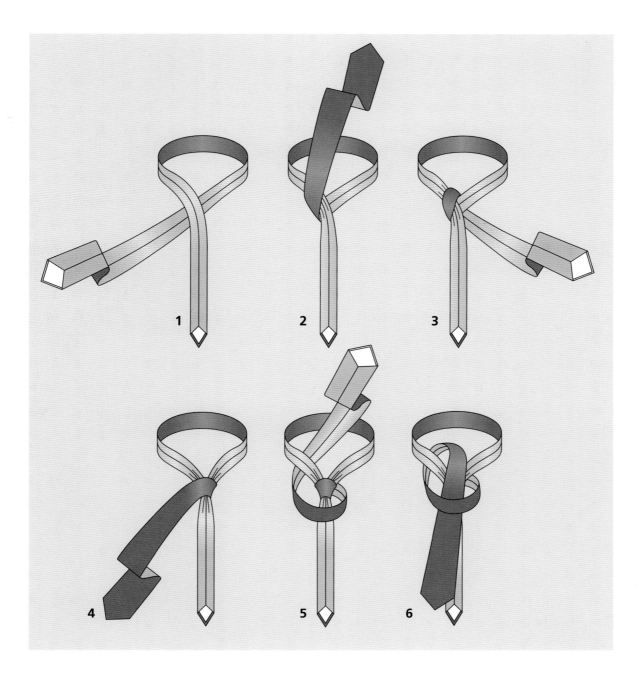

The **PRINCE ALBERT**

The Prince Albert is a derivative of the Four-in-Hand—in fact, it's basically the Four-in-Hand with one extra loop. This means the knot, which must be pulled tight to give it a tidy, slender look, has more bulk. The tie accordingly shortens, meaning it's a great way to go if you're on the shorter side. The Prince Albert works well with narrow-collared shirts. Narrow ties made of softer, more malleable fabrics work best for its configuration.

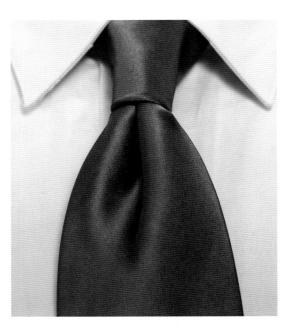

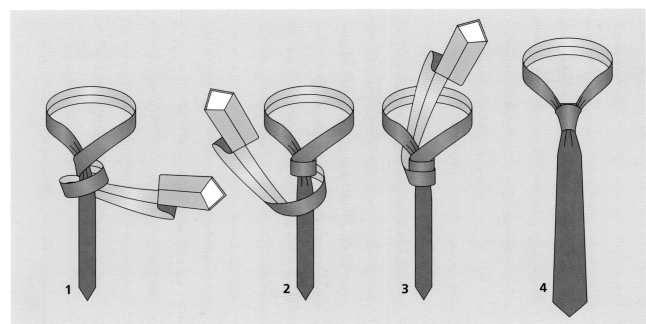

1 2 3 4

The **ORIENTAL**

Sometimes called the "simple knot" and similar to the Four-in-Hand, this tie knot is small and easy to learn. Unlike the Four-in-Hand, though, it is rarely used in the West. As its name suggests, it is China's mainstay tie knot. Give this one a try as a polite, quiet cultural nod or as a subtle way to change your regular Four-in-Hand look. The Oriental's smaller size makes it handy for use with ties of denser fabric and—like all small knots—a good bet if you're on the tall side (the smallness of the tied knot ensures more length left over).

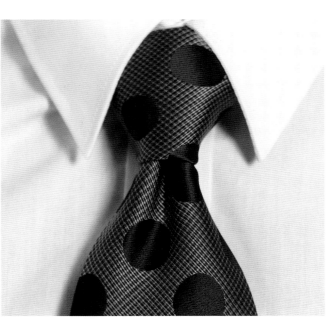

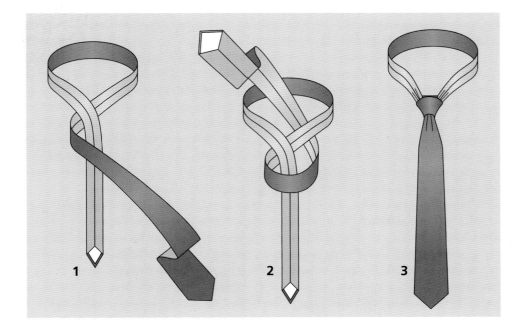

1 **2** **3**

The **CAVENDISH**

The Cavendish knot winds up looking like the ubiquitous Four-in-Hand knot with more presence. It's a large knot, with roughly the same bulk as a Windsor knot, but with a triangular, slightly asymmetrical shape. Unlike some large knots—Windsor included—the Cavendish works well with both spread and narrower collars. It is the youngest of the tie knots, discovered by Fink and Mao in their Cavendish laboratory in the late 1990s. It is slightly more difficult to tie than the others, but we offer it as a good-looking knot that will give you something to do if you've finished your morning coffee and newspaper early. If you're feeling less than dexterous, this will nimble your digits right up.

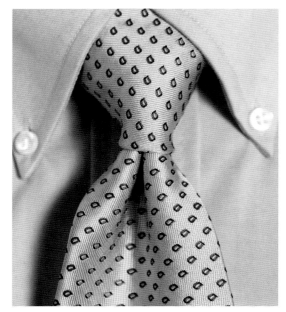

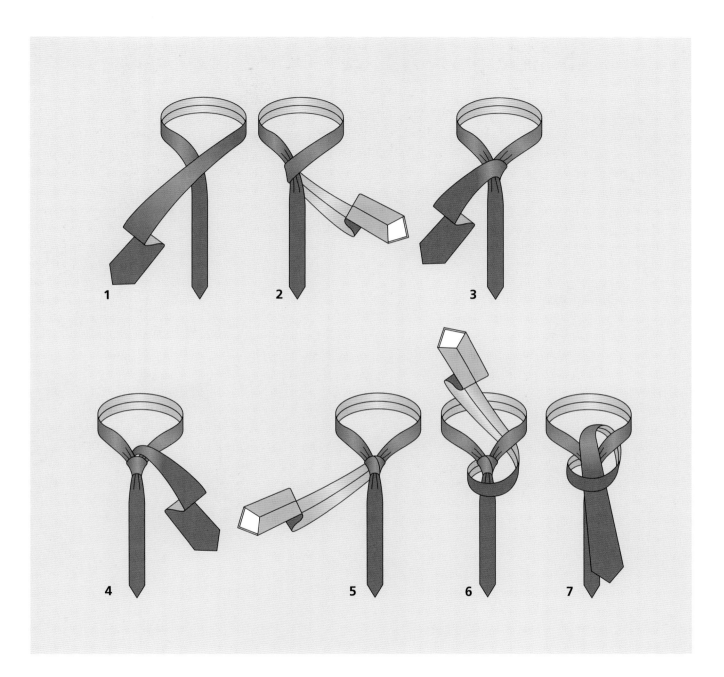

1

2

3

4

5

6

7

The **NICKY**

The Nicky is the invention of the Italian Ernesto Curami of the Nicky tie shop in Milan, though for some time its use was limited to Italy. It returned to the tie-knot lexicon in the late 1980s by accident, when Englishman David Kelsall tied the Pratt the wrong way and got the Nicky instead. The Nicky, which starts inside out like the Oriental, is a medium-sized knot—its classic look goes well with lots of different types of face shapes, tie types, and shirt collars.

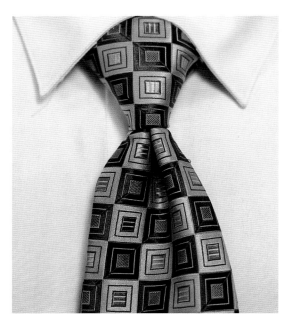

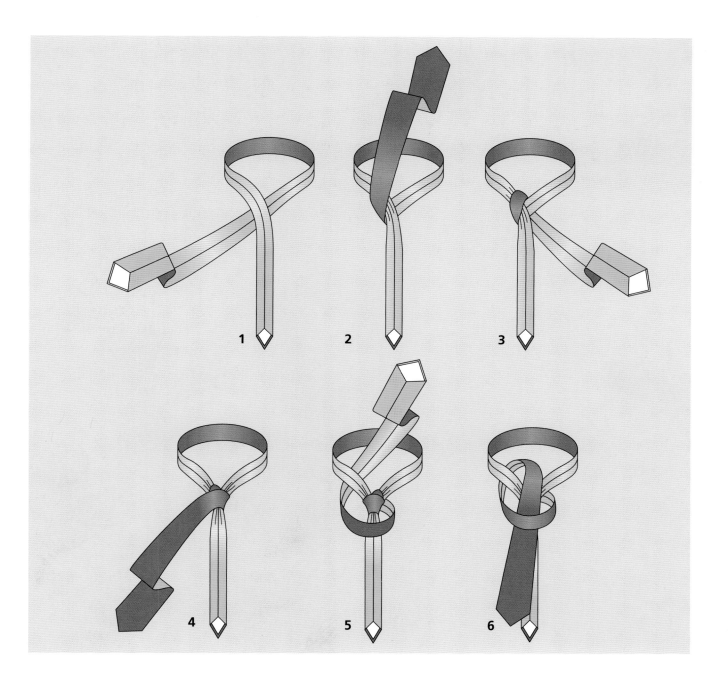

1 2 3

4 5 6

4.
pulling it **OFF**

Style is a simple way of saying complicated things.
JEAN COCTEAU (1889–1963)

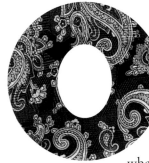 SCAR WILDE NOTED THAT "A WELL-TIED TIE is the first serious step in life," but surely he meant the second step— because no matter your knack for tying a decent knot, if you pair the tie with a shirt that clashes or a jacket whose lapel style wars with the tie's width, what is the point? The point is this: You want to look put together without (a) trying hard to look put together and (b) *looking* like you tried hard to look put together. And this is more likely what Wilde was aiming at, his "well-tied tie" implying the achievement of a well-dressed state, rather than simply the mastery of a Half-Windsor or Four-in-Hand. At the end of the day, most men actually have pretty good instincts about this stuff. The trouble is that at

There's more to the look than simply "tying the knot." Follow your instincts toward choosing pieces that complement each other.

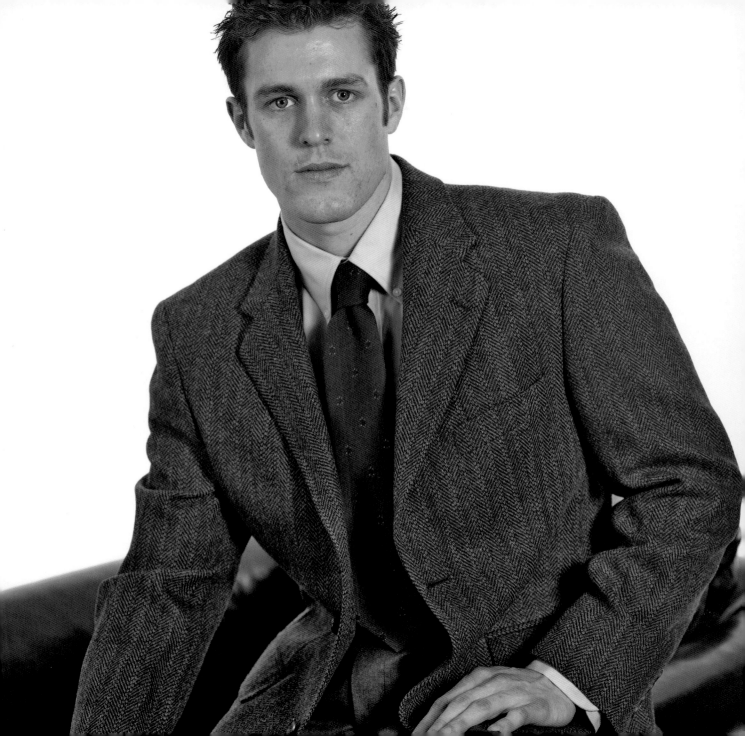

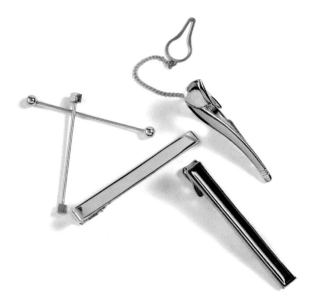

the day's beginning, before that first cup of coffee, most men don't always trust their instincts—or else their instincts, like the rest of them, are groggy or rushed. There's not a man on the planet who, presented with the daily challenge "Which tie goes with which shirt?" hasn't ever fumbled the play. More often than not, the problem is a simple one: You just don't have enough ties, or the right ties, to go with the shirts and/or suits you own. Assembling a solid, basic tie wardrobe that suits your dress needs will eliminate much of the petty angst of last-minute choices.

Along with matching ties to shirts and jackets

to ties, there's a whole little galaxy of tie accessories and complements you'll want to be familiar with: clips, pins, tacks, bars, and pocket squares. Even if you don't plan to actually use any of these accoutrements, it's important to know what they are. You should also know about the rules and regulations of comportment while wearing the actual articles. When, for example, is it unacceptable to wear your tie loosened? You'll find the answer (and to that question, the answer is, "Always") in the information that follows. Mostly, though, we offer suggestions for how to make sure you've got enough ties to mix and match with the shirts and suits or jackets you plan to wear them with as well as parameters and benchmarks for how to coordinate ties with shirts and jackets, employ tie clips and other accessories, and generally wear a tie well. We trust to you take care of the rest nicely.

WHEN to **WEAR** a **TIE**

The number of ties you should own depends on how often you plan or imagine having to wear one. Some business professions mandate their daily wear, though the advent of the 1990s dot-com industry and the related institution of Casual Friday did away with much required tie wear in the business arena and in

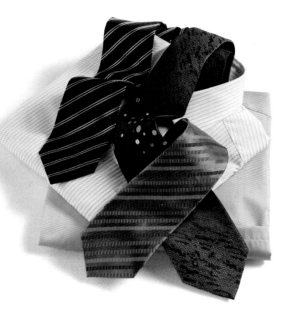

many social scenarios. While the formality of men's professional dress codes has been somewhat revived by the dot-com decline, the rules are now generally more flexible and are best adhered to with a keen eye to local custom and common sense. In other words, a quick survey of the people at the office will tell you when it's okay or not okay to wear a tie.

Social situations lend themselves to slightly less defined do's and don'ts. A handful of types of events and circumstances still require you to wear a tie, such as black-tie functions (see page 78) or those requiring morning dress (see page 84). Some restaurants, men's clubs, and country clubs still require that men and even boys wear a coat and tie and will give you the boot if your clothes don't conform. (Or they'll offer you the dreaded in-house tie and coat reserved for offenders. Those institutions that continue this practice, which has particularly mortified the youngest among us, claim to want to assist those in need, but their intent is clearly propelled by more nefarious motives: punish the forgetful by forcing them to wear grotesque ties and coats in the company of their associates or peers.) Again, most situations require you to decide based on observation and sensibility. If it doesn't feel entirely instinctual 100 percent of the time, you're not alone. The most important thing is to get the lay of the land—West Coast or European notions of when you need to wear a tie may differ at times from East Coast or American—and to wear a tie that you like, that goes with what you're wearing, and that you feel comfortable in. The rest is a piece of cake.

HOW MANY TIES
Do You **NEED**?

On at least one matter, the conventional wisdom of men's style and dress experts is unanimous: Every man must own at least one tie. It's important to get the numbers right: whether one is enough for you, a few will take care of your needs, or your job demands you wear one at least every weekday. Although you can't have too many ties, coming up short is a problem, as it can mean forcing ties with shirts and jackets they don't work with, looking silly and feeling less than confident, and wasting valuable time trying to sort it all out. The information that follows will give you a good idea of how many and what kind of ties you need.

If you're going to own just one tie, make it a solid silk tie in a dark color: charcoal gray, black, navy, or some other dark shade of blue. The most versatile tie is a black knit silk tie, as it can work with a shirt and jeans or a custom-made suit. Versatility, however, is generally overrated. While you might get away with this approach, you run a definite risk of looking like someone who uses versatility as an excuse to be a cheapskate.

Even if you wear ties just now and then, it's best to have a few on hand for different occasions and seasons. A safe handful should include a few solids in dark and/or versatile colors such as red and yellow, some with diagonal or "rep" stripes, and some classic all-over patterns (see page 68). We suggest all silk, with maybe a cotton or wool tie thrown in to mix things up for summer and winter. You may prefer less traditional patterns and colors, in which case adapt accordingly, making sure your existing wardrobe accommodates bolder or more whimsical hues and prints.

If you wear a tie every day, or every workday, you should own at least one tie for each shirt and each suit in your closet. You can get by with a baker's dozen or so, but eventually even this many may leave you repeating your tie/shirt/suit combinations a little too frequently. There's nothing wrong with stepping out in a suit, shirt, and tie combination that looks great with some regularity, but you don't want to be someone who never mixes up his wardrobe. Also, your ties will last longer if they're given a breather between outings. The best solution is to have a couple of ties for each shirt and suit, with each tie affording the ensemble a distinct look. Changing your tie is the easiest, least expensive way to give your style variety

Again, the safe bet is to buy mostly silk ties, with one or two in other natural fabrics, in classic patterns and colors (see page 67). For variety, make the second tie for each shirt and suit a more interestingly hued or unusually patterned version—a subtle floral print in a secondary color or a slightly racier stripe. What you've got in the way of shirts and suits will dictate how adventurous you should be: If your shirts are mostly white or pale, solid colors, you can pair them with lots of different ties, traditional and on the wilder side. Likewise, blue or gray suits can take lots of different ties. If you own a lot of patterned shirts or subtly striped or patterned suits, you'll need to build your tie wardrobe a bit more conservatively.

A **TIE** a **DAY**

Once you've bought well-made ties that you know how to knot and that generally work with the clothes you have, it's time to get down to the real business—which tie to wear with the chosen shirt, jacket, or suit. If you've amassed your tie collection according to our general guidelines and your best instincts, you've won half the battle. A quick perusal of your closet should turn up a tie that will work. Past that, there are just a couple of things you need to consider to leave the house looking great. The tie (and its knot) should work with the shirt collar and jacket or suit style and be suitable to the occasion (formal or casual) and season (cool or warm weather). These considerations determine what fabrics, colors, and patterns—and combinations thereof—are appropriate (see page 67). A good overall rule of thumb is that the elements of any ensemble should never be too disjunctive or too alike. The following sections offer some touchstones to help you get it right.

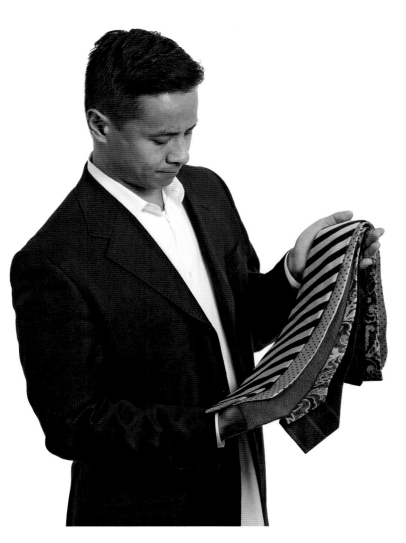

Not all ties make for the appropriate tie-and-shirt combination. Assess your outfit and choose a tie based on its context.

COLLARS and TIES

Before you get into coordinating textures, colors, and patterns, there are a couple rules to matching the tie with jacket lapels and shirt collars.

Buying ties in the standard dimensions described in Chapter 2 will more or less ensure that your tie is appropriate for your jacket lapel. The width of the tie should always match the width of the lapel: standard tie with standard lapel, wider tie with wide lapel, thinner tie with thin lapel, and so on.

Many types of shirt collars are worn for casual, professional, and formal wear. Ties should only be worn with certain shirt collars, and some knots work better with some shirt collars than with others. The fabric and length of the tie you choose to wear will affect to some degree how well it works with a particular shirt collar. Finding which of your ties works best with a particular shirt may take some trial and error, but here is some general guidance.

Button-Down

This is the old standby, with collar points that button to the shirt. If you wear it with a tie, use one of the bigger knots, such as a Windsor.

Straight or Point

The points of this collar are longer than the points of other collars, though different versions come in different lengths. This shirt looks great with a tie and works well with any tie knot—small, medium, or slightly bulky.

Tab

The tab that shows between the collar's points means that this type of shirt is always worn with a tie. The tab supports the tie and gives it a more formal look. Only a small knot, such as the Four-in-Hand, will work.

Spread

The gap between this collar's points is wider and the collar itself is stiffer than the straight collar. It should always be worn with a larger tie, such as one with a Half- or Full Windsor knot. A British spread is a more formal version of the spread collar. The British spread should always be worn with a tie featuring a larger knot, such as a Windsor, to fill the gap between its points.

Banded

This shirt has no collar. It should therefore never be worn with a tie.

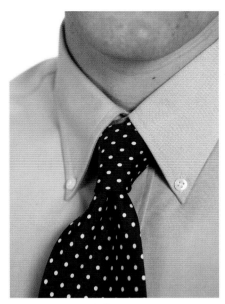

Button-Down Collar

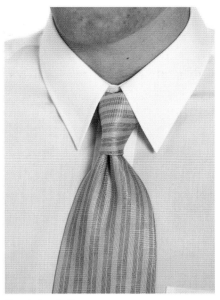

Straight Collar

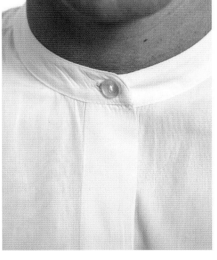

Banded Collar

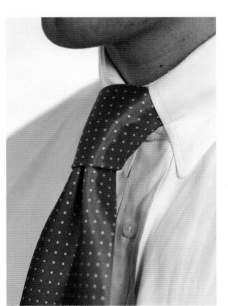

Tab Collar

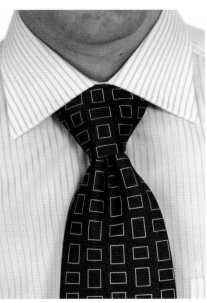

Spread Collar

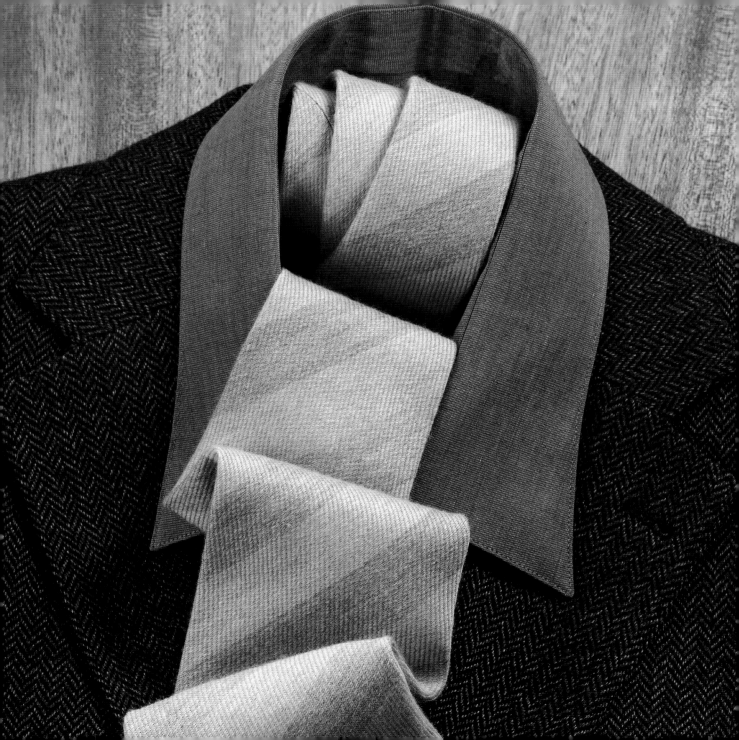

COORDINATING TIES, SHIRTS, and JACKETS:
Fabric, Color, and Pattern

There is no exact science to coordinating a particular tie with a particular shirt or jacket. Instinct and practice (and the confirmation of success by loved ones and colleagues) will be your best mentors. But even the best instinct can—when confronted with too little time to decide, an unfamiliar circumstance, or just a bad day—go awry. The following collective tips will help keep instinct on the straight and narrow.

Fabric

Different fabrics denote more or less formality, and ties made from them should be worn accordingly. A good rule of thumb is that the softer the fabric, the fancier the tie. A woven silk tie is as formal as a straight tie gets; printed silk, depending on the pattern, can work with less formal or casual looks. A more rough-textured fabric, such as wool, cotton, or linen, is better for wear with a more casual jacket and shirt. The key is to make sure the tone of the shirt, jacket, and tie fabrics are in accord. A rough tweed jacket won't look good with an extremely fine-woven silk tie; a substantial winter suit doesn't work with a lightweight cotton tie; and a luxe silk suit shouldn't be paired with a nubby knitted wool tie.

Color

Common sense and a good look at the world around you will tell you much about which colors should and should not be allowed to congregate. Gone are the days when certain colors were absolute no-can-do's for certain seasons (or, for that matter, for men), but that's not to say it's open season for color collaboration. Only guys with a highly instinctual or honed faculty for style can pull off anarchic color combinations, and they're relatively few and far between. Some of what you need to know is pretty obvious: Darker, muted hues better suit serious, more formal occasions and are an obvious choice for fall and winter wear. Brighter, bolder colors are better for warm-weather seasons and for more casual or celebratory goings-on. Pastels, neutrals, and earth tones are flexible and can look casual or very elegant. The easiest ways to color-match ties with shirts and jackets is to coordinate the shirt to one of the tie's colors, preferably one that's dominant in the tie and contrasts with the shirt, or choose the tie that has the greatest amount of the color you want to emphasize in your shirt and jacket.

On the other hand, unless you're expressly going for a monochromatic look—solid-colored tie on same-color solid shirt (this works in some cases)—focusing too much on one

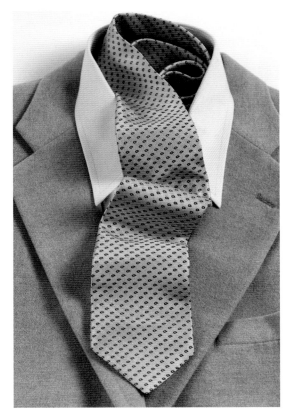

Pattern

Coordinating shirt and tie patterns is the most difficult aspect of choosing a tie. As the saying goes: If at first you don't succeed, try, try again (and don't leave the house until you're sure you've got it right). There is no foolproof advice in this matter, but stick with these basic tenets and you'll be fine.

Generally speaking, motifs get more formal as they get smaller—a diminutive dot or subtle stripe is automatically fancier than a big dot or bold stripe. The easiest approach to successfully wearing a patterned tie is to pair it with a solid shirt—or pair a solid tie with a patterned shirt. But life, as we know from countless parental lectures in our youth, is not easy. And if there's adventure to be had in the daily routine of tie choosing, surely it's your due. In other words, you'll want to mix it up a little, and that's fine. Just do it with care. When you combine patterns, pay attention to pattern similarity and contrast, their relative scale, and type. You can mix patterns; for example, dots and stripes can work together but only if the patterns' scales are similar. The reverse is true when you're wearing a shirt and tie that share a basic pattern: A striped tie will look good with a striped shirt only if the stripes are different sizes or widths. In this vein, make sure that

color can make you look staid or drab. What works best is contrasting a primary color with a secondary color in its family—red with orange, say, or blue with purple—or contrasting two colors that complement each other, such as navy and burgundy or blue and orange. That way, you wind up with a look that's lively but not brash.

same-sized patterns don't "track" each other—that is, run catercorner to each other in the ensemble so that the effect is of a basket weave. Except on fashion runways, busy patterns are never to be seen in the intimate company of other busy patterns. Don't pair wild Escheresque geometric prints with splashy flowered shirts, for example.

TIE ACCESSORIES

Accessories for straight ties comprise a small group that should be managed with care. A good tie doesn't need any bells and whistles, and each clip, tack, bar, and chain will more likely than not make it a less fashionable tie. There are exceptions, and you'll find them—along with general information on tie accessories—noted below.

Tie Clips, Pins, and Chains

All of these accessories are intended to serve the same purpose: keeping the tie in place. Tiepins got their start in the early 1800s, keeping the many folds of elaborately tied ascots anchored. Initially simple unadorned pins, they became more extravagant as fashions changed over the centuries and now exist in conservative, elaborate, and whimsical versions. A tie tack—a shorter version with a

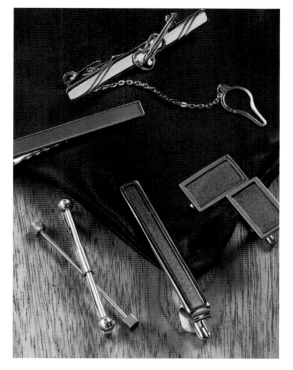

pinch-clasp backing—is a more modern rendition of the tiepin. Both are dated, and both poke tiny but permanent holes in your tie. Although some menswear specialists suggest that a tie chain anchors the tie and hangs "decoratively" across the front of the tie, too much accessory is simply tacky. In a sense, tie chains are to ties what a chinstrap is to a hat.

The one tie-securing option that can look good is a tie clip, a small oblong bar worn very low on the tie with a clip on the back that holds the tie in place. Be careful when picking one out, because some have small rows of teeth that can cut into and damage your tie. Go with a vintage sterling one, and steer clear of the new-fangled tie clip "fashions," which are out of fashion as soon as they've arrived.

Pocket Squares

Pocket squares—small, handkerchief squares of fabric made especially for suit-jacket pockets—list to the anachronistic side these days, but both older and younger men still sometimes wear them, and both can make the wearer look good. Some, such as traditional handkerchiefs tucked in the pocket, are white, so matching them to the tie isn't a concern.

A colored pocket square should work with but not be identical to the tie's color and pattern, and it should have a texture that is different from but complementary to the tie. Most natural fabrics—silk, cotton, linen, wool—will work well in this subtle opposition.

The pocket square should be tucked in loosely, not carefully folded, and only a thin part should show above the pocket.

TIE ETIQUETTE

There are many activities a man may appropriately engage in while wearing a tie—some obligatory, some chosen; some arduous, some effortless; some tedious, some fun filled; some modest, some racy. However, there are also a few things a man should never do while wearing a tie, and a survey of popular conduct indicates that more assistance in these matters is required. Here are the rules:

▸ No tie tucking. This means no tucking the tie into the waist of the pants or behind the belt buckle. It means no tucking the narrow side of the tie into the gap between the shirt's buttons. Likewise, when driving a car, the seatbelt goes under the tie so the tie isn't creased after the ride.

▸ No tie tossing. This refers to the loose-noose look favored by certain diners who, rather than being extra careful while eating, make an effort to toss the tie back around the neck, as if in a breezy, devil-may-care moment of insouciance. Instead they look as sloppy as the spill they're trying to avoid.

▸ No tie loosening. This means that unless you are at home, in the process of removing the tie, it should not be in a loosened state. Either leave it on or take it off (where no one can see). Wearing a tie with the knot loosened just looks sloppy.

Pocket squares add fashionable flair to the ordinary suit jacket–tie duo.

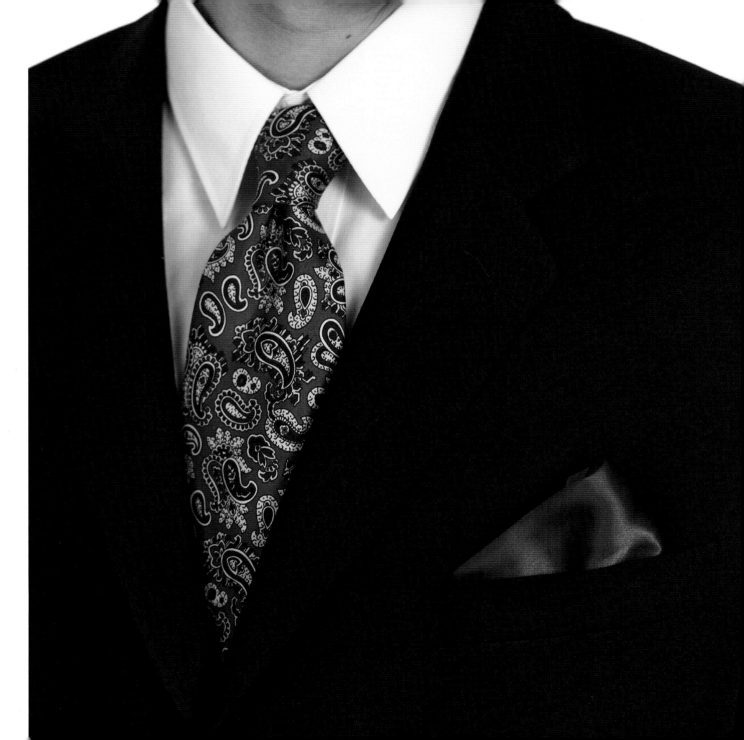

5.
the **BOW** tie

A man is worth as much as his tie—that is, through it he displays his character, in it he manifests his spirit.

HONORÉ DE BALZAC (1799–1850)

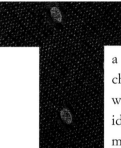

HE BOW TIE IS A TRICKY BIT OF BUSINESS, no two ways about it. For black-tie it's a must, which is why you must know how to choose it, tie it properly, and carry it off. But where everyday wear is concerned, it is the idiosyncratic uncle of the tie world. Make no mistake: Sporting a bow tie will mark you as an individualist and thus garner either or both the admiration and criticism that individualistic acts inspire. The wearing of a bow tie should not be taken lightly, nor is its wearing for the faint of heart. Great men and fools alike have made it emblematic of their endeavors, but there's not much middle ground. It stands out. You get noticed in it. Make sure this is what you want.

Regardless of your inspiration or motivation for donning the bow tie, it is a sure bet for making a statement.

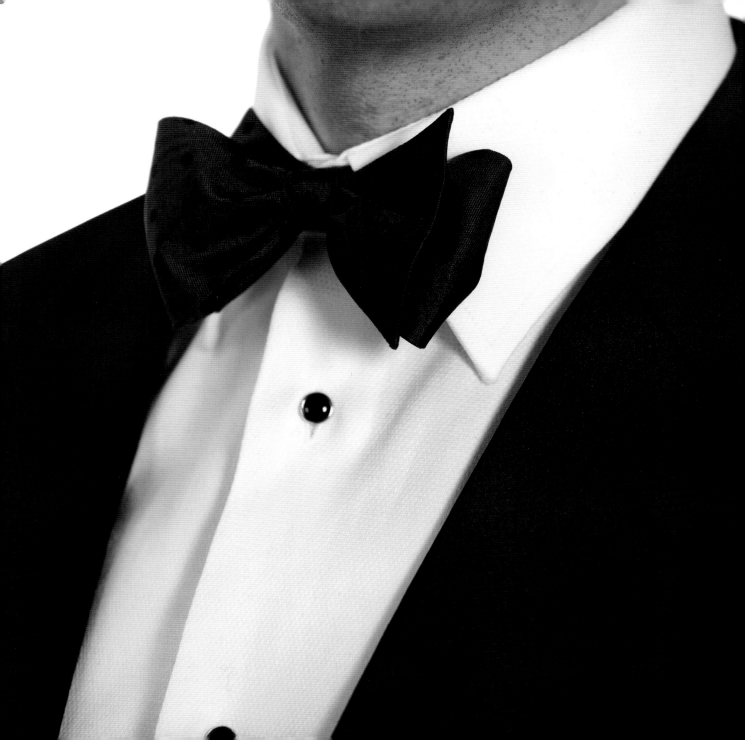

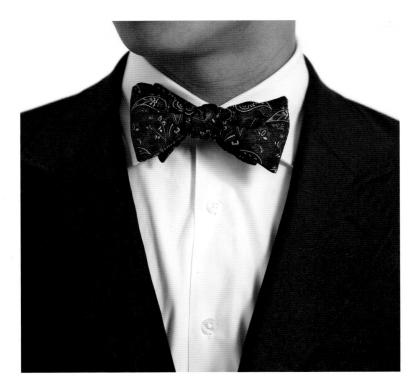

that decade, you may have been forced to wear one to your birthday party.) At that point in history, wearing a bow tie was no big deal.

These days, it's something of a big deal. In order to not look silly while you're wearing one—whether you're going to a wedding or gala, or trying the bow-tie look as a regular thing—you need to know some basic things about the bow tie: how it's made, what good ones are made of, how to tie one, and what to wear it with.

FABRIC

Like straight ties, bow ties may be made of a variety of fabrics. Also like straight ties, they should be purchased for wear in very few of these fabrics. Woven and printed silk, cotton, wool, and certain natural blends make fine bow ties that weather the years and maintain their attractiveness. Other fabrics bring us to the vast overlap between bow tie and novelty tie. There are few among us unfamiliar with the squirting bow tie and its spiritual twin, the spinning bow tie. There are more where these come from: bow ties that light up and flash lights by which to do "The Hustle"; bow ties that light up spelling "HELLO" and other greetings; bow ties carved of wood or molded of acrylic and embedded with objects—fishing flies and paper clips. This is extreme wear for

Like the straight tie, the bow tie is descended from the cravat. It really came into play at the close of the nineteenth century, when it existed in umpteen forms, big and small: stiff, floppy, geometric, loopy, regular, off-center, and more. A walk down a London street during that era would have shown you gentlemen's bow ties tied in any of a dozen or so types of knots. In 1904 a fairly standard bow tie, called the butterfly tie, came onto the scene, more or less to stay. (Those of you who recall the 1970s will remember a large-bow bow tie also known as a butterfly tie. If you were preadolescent during extreme people. But for those of us who are less extreme, it's best to stick to the more standard fabrics. (For more detailed information about tie fabrics, see page 23.)

PATTERN

As with fabric, many of the general rules regarding solids, prints, and patterns outlined in Chapter 2 apply to bow ties, too. Bow ties may be patterned with just about any motif, but the most common patterns are stripes, dots, club prints, geometrics, madras plaid, and tartan plaid. But whatever the rule for straight-tie patterns, it holds doubly true for bow-tie patterns. Most important: Large-motif patterns are nearly impossible to pull off; flora (particularly of the tropical variety) and fauna are too. Though some deviation from the rule is okay, solid colors are the norm for formal wear: black with tux, white with tails (see page 78).

DIMENSIONS

Bow ties have been made and worn in nearly every imaginable smaller-than-a-breadbox dimension but now come in three shapes—two of which are more common—and a more or less standard size. The least common is the smaller and narrowest version, called a "straight" or "thistle" bow tie, which has ends extending straight out on either side, usually straight but

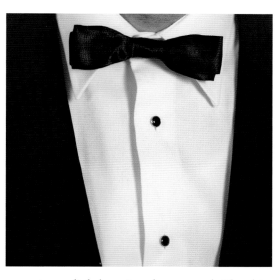

sometimes slightly pointed or curved. The thistle bow tie is just for casual wear. The two commonly worn styles are the "bat" or "bat's wing" and the "butterfly." The butterfly bow tie is the standard, with a more cinched waist and two bow ends that look like two small triangles (hence the moniker). The bat's-wing bow tie has pointed edges, is a little smaller, and is quite a bit narrower than the butterfly. Both are worn for casual and formal wear, though the butterfly shape is most common for black tie. There are no hard-and-fast rules for bow ties vis-à-vis their dimensions. But there are some guidelines to follow.

You don't want it too big or too small. Just as a big, oversized butterfly bow tie will make you look like Bozo the Clown, a mincing little version will make you look like Porky Pig.

The bow tie should not be broader than your neck. When worn, the bow ends should not reach as far as the points of your shirt collar, or the width of your eyes.

Most bow ties, whether bat or butterfly style, are a standard size. If yours is in this range, you're good to go. If it's much bigger or smaller, hand it back to the tailor.

TYPES

Bow ties, like straight ties, come in three forms: the kind you tie yourself, the kind that are pretied, and the ones that are clipped on. You should tie it yourself, and you will learn to do so shortly (see page 80). It's hard, but you'll learn after a few attempts. Wearing a hand-tied bow tie makes it clear you know what you're about. Wearing a ready-tied bow tie is acceptable in a pinch. Wearing a clip-on is never acceptable, unless you're trying to be funny. If you wear it when you're not trying to be funny, you'll still be funny—just to other people, not yourself.

CASUAL Wear

It's difficult to offer much advice beyond what cannot be said strongly enough: Beware. Extremely touchy fashion terrain ahead. Proceed with caution. The man who manages to wear the bow tie with complete success is a king of style: bold, utterly sure of himself, and, it must be said, rare.

For casual wear, a bow tie can be worn with different types of collars but works best with a button-down shirt. The bow tie must be hand tied. That said, in lieu of further strict counsel, we offer up some following considerations.

Bow ties don't dangle or fall forward and therefore don't get in the way. This is why, historically, dentists, doctors, and scientists have opted to wear them. Likewise, they are less likely to be splashed with soup or sauce.

They are lightweight and cover only a very small area. If you wear one in summer or in the tropics, you'll feel cooler than men wearing straight ties. They can increase the import of your originality and authority. They can and will set you apart from the crowd. They can add a festive, celebratory effect to an ensemble.

More food for thought: The artists, political leaders, and men listed below either got away having worn a bow tie or they didn't because they lacked understanding of some or all of the above-listed considerations.

▸ Fifteenth U.S. President Abraham Lincoln: Yes

▸ Early twentieth-century French architect Le Corbusier: Yes

▸ Spanish poet Federico García Lorca: Yes

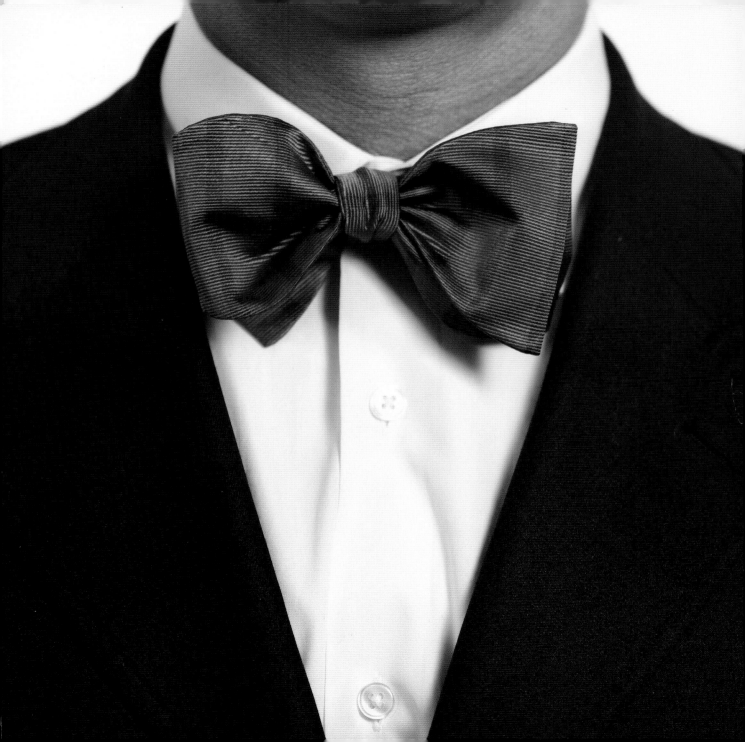

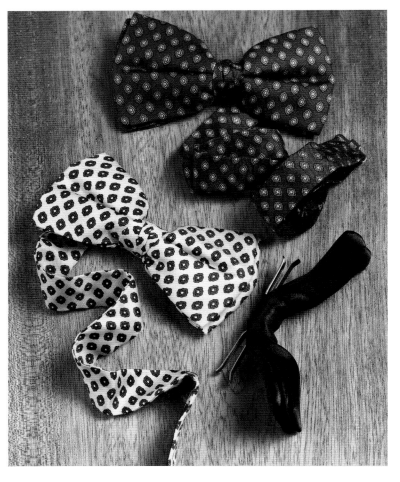

- ▸ British Prime Minister Sir Winston Churchill: Yes
- ▸ Entertainer and all-around style slickster Frank Sinatra: Yes
- ▸ Phonograph inventor Thomas Edison: Yes
- ▸ Irish playwright and quipster Oscar Wilde: Yes

- ▸ Mariachis: Yes
- ▸ Thirty-third U.S. President Harry S. Truman: No
- ▸ Apple computer founder Steve Jobs: No
- ▸ Junior conservative pundit and minor television celeb Tucker Carlson: No
- ▸ Junior pundits, generally: No
- ▸ Juniors, generally (see above, Steve Jobs and Tucker Carlson): No
- ▸ Pundits, generally: No
- ▸ Arts critic Gene Shalit: Resoundingly, no
- ▸ Barney Fife from *The Andy Griffith Show*: No

FORMAL Wear
Black Ties and White Ties

A black bow tie is imperative for every man's wardrobe: a necessity for wear with a tuxedo for black-tie events. Even if you rent the tux (which you should not if you attend two or more black-tie events a year), you should own the bow tie. It must be silk or brocade and hand-tied. If it's not black, keep it dark—navy or deep midnight blue.

Some men feel that wearing a black tie for black-tie events leaves them feeling like just one more penguin in the group. Thus, some men opt for patterned bow ties for black-tie wear. Almost without exception, this makes them look like just one particularly unfortunate penguin in the group. Patterns that can work are elegant stripes, minuscule checks or dots, or subtle paisley. For extremely formal occasions requiring white-tie dress, you'll need a white tie. This degree of formality is rarely required nowadays, and most men don't own the elements of white-tie attire: tailcoat, waistcoat, top hat, scarf and gloves, and tie. If you need these for a special occasion, they are available for rent.

Cummerbunds, Suspenders, and Cuff Links

It's simple: The cummerbund matches the bow tie in color and material. The cummerbund should be worn with the pleats pointing upward, as the cummerbund used to be employed as a ticket holder for theatergoers. The suspenders, if worn, do not clip on; they have buttonholes and are attached with buttons. They also match the bow tie and cummerbund. Cuff links round out the formal wear accessory list and look best in silver, gold, or black onyx. Keep them discreet and elegant in style. Heirloom or sought-after vintage numbers, if worn well, can be a big hit.

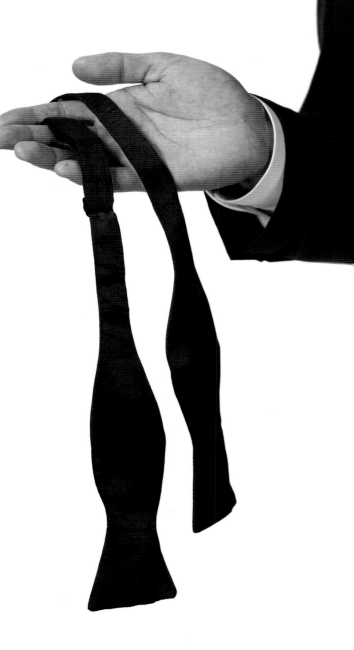

TYING It

Wear a poorly tied bow tie and you look as though you've had one too many, even if the party hasn't yet begun. As previous sections of this chapter have noted, something about the slightly eccentric nature of a bow tie means that wearing one can stand you on the precipice of sartorial success or disaster. Once you've made sure the quality, color, pattern, and shape of your bow tie are the right stuff, what remains is the matter of how you tie and wear it. Your comportment is, of course, ultimately up to you. But the knowledge that you're properly put together goes a long way to feeling confident, particularly on more important occasions requiring a black tie.

It's worth spending the time to learn how to tie a bow tie correctly. It will take a few attempts and may be slightly frustrating. But your rewards will be reaped in the form of less sweat when a last-minute formal event presents itself, and the conviction that when you appear at a business function, the boss doesn't think you're wearing a pretied or clip-on bow tie.

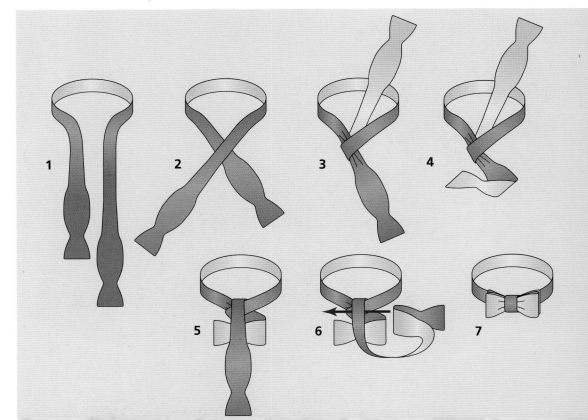

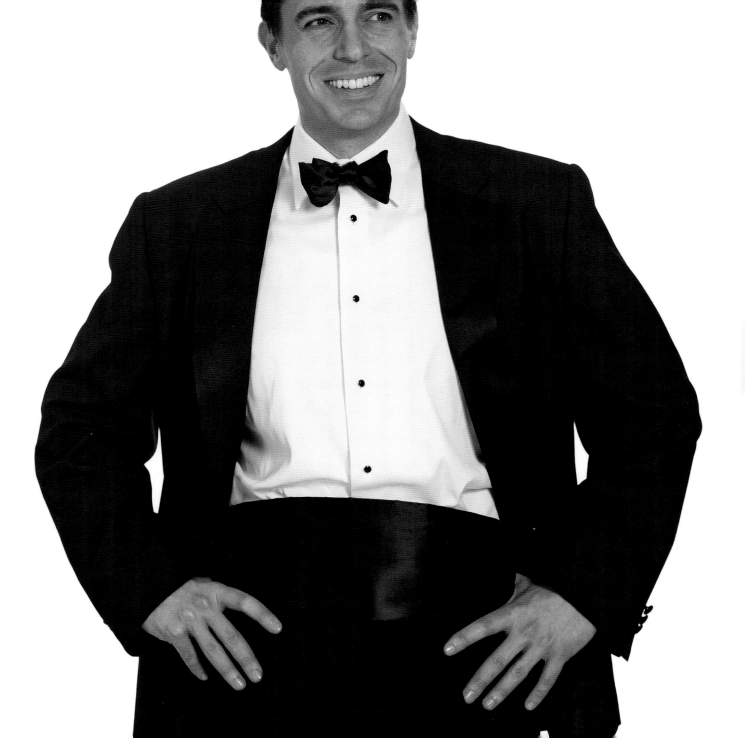

6.
the **ASCOT** and other anomalies

The fact that I arrive at the office every morning wearing an ordinary striped tie is significant, as is my replacing it on a whim with a psychedelic tie, or my attending a business meeting without wearing a tie at all.

UMBERTO ECO, *Psychology of Clothes*, 1972

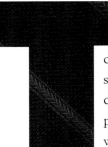

THE KIND OF TIE YOU CHOOSE TO WEAR says a lot about you. You may never consider wearing anything but a straight-up straight tie, and that may well be the best style choice you ever make. W. Somerset Maugham put it this way: "The well-dressed man is he whose clothes you never notice." And, as is true with dinner party conversation or workplace chitchat, less is more with regard to what tie you wear. You're more likely to win friends and influence people by saying less (rather than too much) about yourself and your fashion sense. In this vein, not surprisingly there exists some striking common ground between a man in an ascot, bola tie, string tie, or novelty tie and a man who tirelessly name-drops or can't keep quiet. In other words,

Although most men are familiar and comfortable with the traditional necktie, you may find purpose in and derive pleasure from deviations such as the ascot.

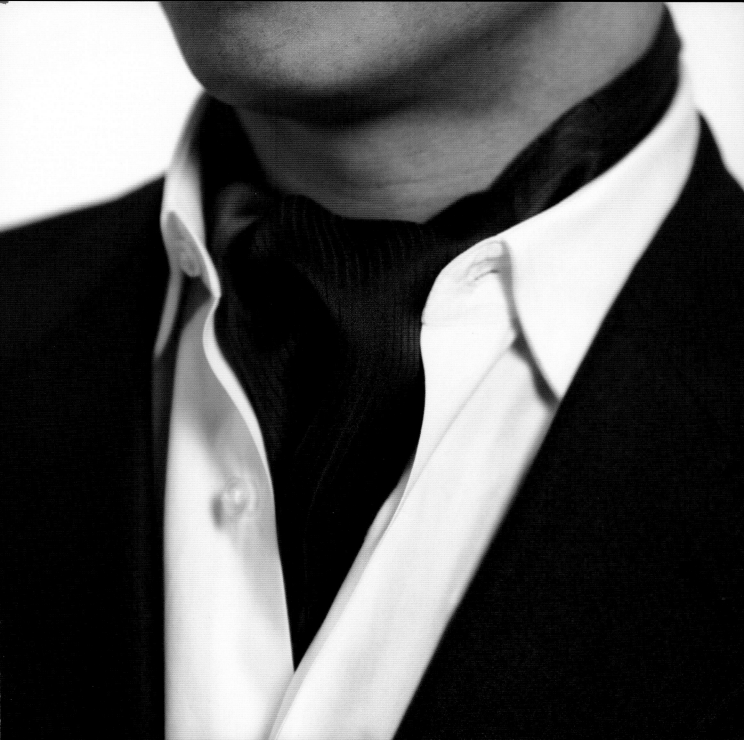

these are neckwear choices made by men who don't mind saying "Look at me." They're choices that have to do with attitude.

Now that the red flag has been firmly hoisted, you're wondering: Why should I care? Well, that's the point. Maybe you shouldn't. As Gore Vidal wrote, "Style is knowing who you are, what to say, and not giving a damn." And here's the rub: Not a few titans of industry and the arts have made their marks by successfully stepping out with some style attitude, and we like to think that the readers of this book include just some such men.

That is not to suggest to land the cover of *Forbes* or to find your way to history's centerfold you need to wear an eccentric tie. For those who will stick with the straight tie, let this chapter serve as entertaining arcane. If you like a little retro in your look but don't want to go the bow-tie route, this section on vintage ties will give you some handy tips.

ASCOT

The ascot is basically a smallish scarf worn loosely tied around the neck and tucked into a shirt, taking its name from England's renowned Royal Ascot horse racing event, at which it was once required wear for male attendees, along with top hat and tails. It is a type of cravat and was very popular in the latter part of the nineteenth century among members of the middle and upper classes, when it was most often worn with a tiepin to keep it in place. The advent of the straight tie slowly but surely rendered the ascot all but extinct in the menswear menagerie. (Note: Ascots are still commonly referred to as cravats, though in fact "cravat" may be used to refer to any type of neckwear.)

There are, in fact, certain rare functions (the occasional fancy daytime wedding, the odd Ascot-or-equivalent horse race) for which the ascot is still required wear, as it is part of traditional "morning dress" and thus worn with top hat and tails. Unlike a tux, no one expects you to own your own garments for morning dress; if you find yourself in need, hurry down to a serious men's outfitter or formal-wear shop and rent them. The shop's staff will help you figure out how to tie the ascot, or you can go with the ready-tied version.

On the subject of wearing the ascot casually, we offer the ensuing sequence of observations and considerations:

Men who get away with wearing an ascot tend to be arrestingly handsome (see Cary Grant), devilishly charming (see David Niven), or iconically astute (see Sherlock Holmes).

Behold the Neck Slip, the bygone necktie-ascot hybrid.

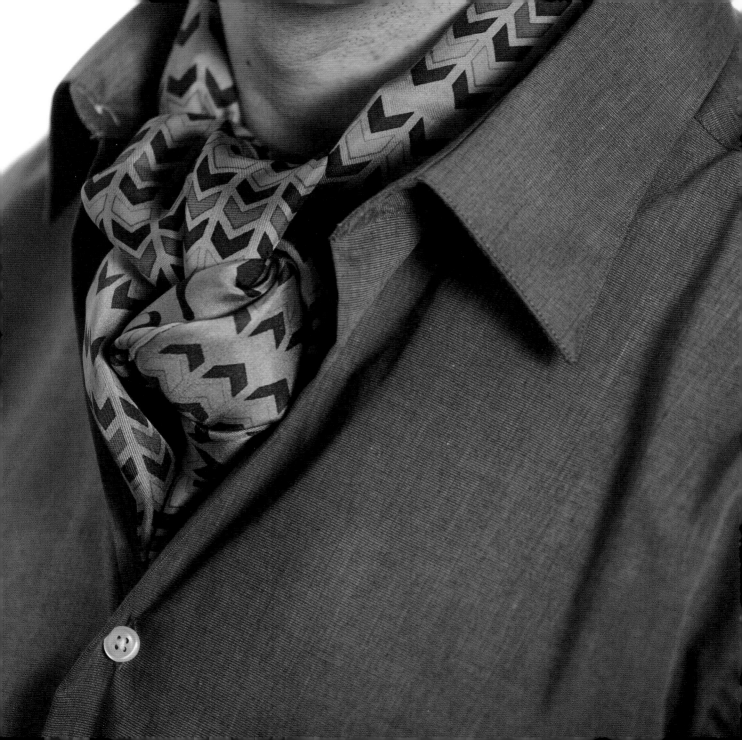

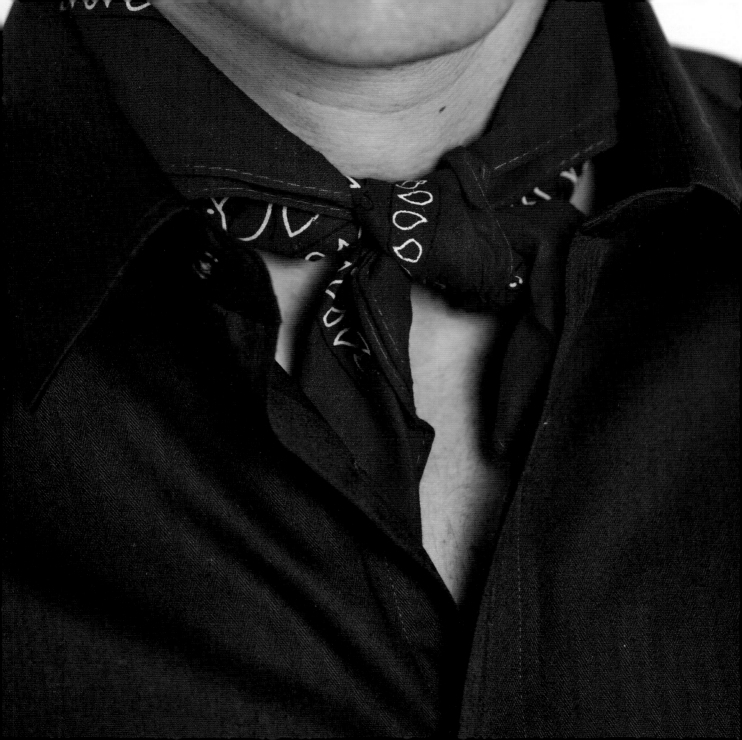

Men who get away with wearing an ascot are almost always over the age of forty-five, usually with at least some dignified silver in their hair (see any man under the age of forty-five wearing an ascot).

NECK SLIP

The neck slip is an esoteric hybrid of the straight tie and the ascot. It is worn looped and tucked in a very loose knot, with the front, arrow-shaped end tucked into the front of the shirt. Usually seen in the vicinity of a velvet smoking jacket with sateen lapels and an ebony cigarette holder, the neck slip seems to be relegated to bygone stars and directors of horror movies and their present-day camp worshippers. The most recent sighting is believed to have been on Vincent Price at a series of Hollywood poolside cocktail parties, circa 1957 to 1962.

BANDANA

We think of the bandana as a totem of the American West, but the word *bandana* is actually Sanskrit. Imported to England from India and the States in the early eighteenth century, the bandana started out as a silk kerchief in vivid Indian hues. It was the first brightly colored necktie to be worn among Westerners. Gradually, for reasons of practicality and expense, it evolved into the better-known cotton form we know today. Though it's most often thought of in conjunction with cowboys, early railroad workers, or other American pioneers, it actually got its first stateside play sported by a boxer named James Belcher. Perhaps because of its working-class origins and more man-of-the-street associations, the bandana—though often worn in much the same way as the ascot—doesn't as readily shriek pretentiousness as an ascot does. If you want to try out the look, wear it with a cotton shirt and knot it like a kerchief or cross and tuck it loosely like an ascot.

BOLA (BOLO)

The bola tie, also referred to as a bolo tie, was invented by an Arizona cowboy named Vic Cedarstaff. The story goes that some time in the 1940s, Vic was on the range, and his hat blew away. The hat, like most cowboy hats, was encircled at the point where the crown joins the brim by a leather or suede cord held in place by a metal clasp of sorts. When our man Vic recovered the hat, he took the cord and clasp and strung them around his neck to keep them safe. Back at the ranch, other cowboys copied the look, and it stuck. (Note: "Bola" is Spanish for two-ended lassos, favored by Argentine cowboys for

The Bandana: Not just for cowboys.

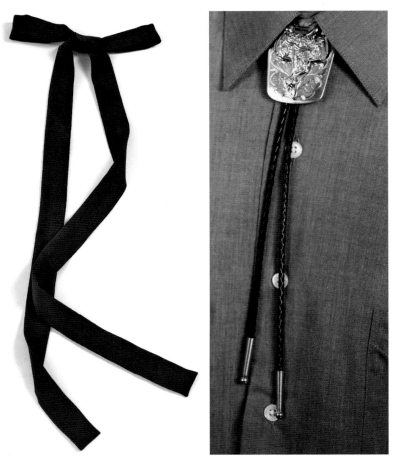

Left: **String Tie**; *Right:* **Bola**

of cotton or velvet tied so that its longish ends hang over the top of the wearer's chest. Elvis worked the look pretty well, but that was another time and he was Elvis. Interestingly British Teddy boys fancied the look and wore string ties they called Slim Jims with their drainpipe pants and snarky, tough-guy pouts.

NOVELTY TIES

There are only two ways the novelty tie should be worn: as a clear and present joke or an unmistakable caper, such as to a costume party; or with a style sensibility that cleverly manages to incorporate the tie as an ironic footnote to some slick, toned-down getup. Problem: As with the novelty theme tie, the novelty tie—which may be made of just about any material and can vary greatly in shape and size—is only for the courageous. In other words, men who wear novelty ties mistakenly wear them either without humor or with entirely the wrong brand of humor.

VINTAGE

Since tie-design pioneer Jesse Langsdorf patented the bias-cut tie in the 1920s, the straight tie's nonstructural qualities—width, shape, color, and pattern styles—have fluctuated over the decades. Like other changing fashion trends—women's necklines, for instance—the shifts have been sometimes subtle and some-

catching wild horses.) The bola tie has been the official tie of Arizona since 1971.

STRING

Like most things that have been caricaturized, the string tie started out more or less as a southern version of a bow tie—a narrow strip

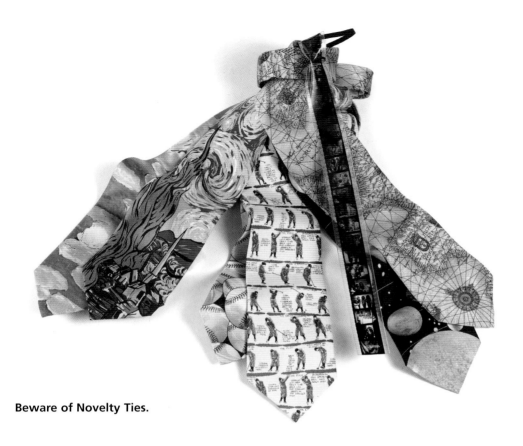

Beware of Novelty Ties.

times drastic. At least some men must have cared well for their ties in bygone times, because you can still find other-era ties to wear today.

Vintage ties—particularly those from the 1920s through the mid-1950s—can look great if you find or inherit ones that are good looking and in good shape. Older male relatives' closets and attic boxes, along with vintage and thrift stores, flea markets, and yard sales, can cough up some very cool ties that, worn with the right shirt and/or jacket, can give your look a little edge without making you look like you tried too hard. Silk and other natural fibers—cotton, wool, and blends—or rayon are the way to go, and it's key to make sure the tie width approximates the width of the jacket you want to wear it with. The following sections offer a few pointers to help you discern which era you're dealing with.

The 1920s

Ties in the 1920s were celebrated for their resilience, in no small part due to Langsdorf's landmark design patent. As throughout most of history, silk was the fabric of choice. Knit ties, which resurface every couple of decades (and perennially hold their own fairly well) were very trendy and came in a bevy of shapes, sizes, and forms—two-toned, reversible, and tight, loose, and specialty-weave knits. Darker hues were fashionable: dark reds and off-reds, purples, navy and midnight blues, browns, and blacks. Diagonally striped or rep ties were particularly popular.

The 1930s

This decade witnessed the birth and growth of Hollywood and the movie biz, so too the fashion focus was directed to what Hollywood stars and starlets were wearing. Likewise, the famously elegant Duke of Windsor's stateside trip drew attention to men's dress and ties in particular—the duke was a devil for a properly tied tie (though not tied in a Windsor knot; see page 46).

Gangster fashion also took hold to some degree in certain man-on-the-street ranks. The result of these diverse influences was a mix of tie styles that ranged from tidy and

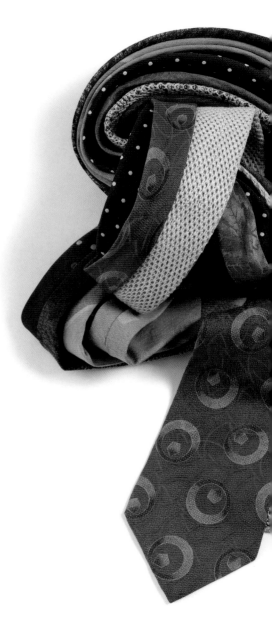

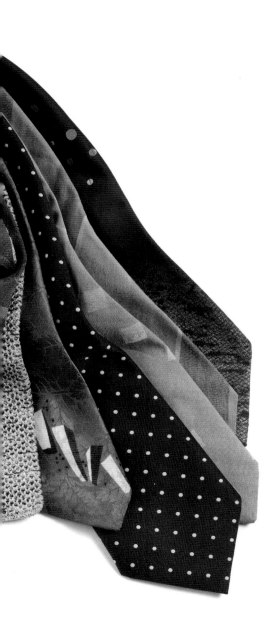

conservative to flashy and wild. Ties came in silk, satin, and blended weaves and increasingly in rayon, which was cheaper, more resistant to spots and tears, and easier to clean. Solid ties were popular but myriad eclectic prints big and small also flourished—bold and subtle checks, stripes, all-overs, and other patterns. By the late 1930s, new weaving techniques and fabrics made for more intricate and complicated prints. Patterns of flora, fauna, abstract and geometric designs, and stylized plumes and swirls were common. This era also produced what might be called the first novelty ties, ties with individualized or advertising slogans.

The 1940s and 1950s

This period was a tie heyday, as economic conservatism necessitated by World War II had a huge impact on tie production and tie-design evolution. A greatly reduced number of ties were actually manufactured, but tie makers with more time on their hands dreamed up a pantheon of new looks for ties. Along with the many types of colors and patterns the 1930s had ushered in came a new look based on an emerging Art Deco palette and graphics, and patterns became increasingly abstract and/or geometric. The tie's postwar color and pattern schemes were celebratory. Ties came in bright colors and wild, fun, even outrageous patterns with motifs larger than ever before: bold contrasting vertical stripes; highly stylized plumes, petals, birds, and other nature icons; themes with tropical, Asian, Middle Eastern, Cubist-inspired, and American West motifs; images of everything from cards to roadsters, flamingos to Parisian street scenes, cowboys to spaceships.

In 1947 *Esquire* defined this as the "bold look," which characterized the tie through the mid-1950s. During the "bold look" reign, ties were largely made of Dacron and rayon, with a wide range of new weaving techniques and printing methods, including hand painting, screen printing, and even photographic processes. The late 1950s toned the tie down again; ties became more conservative, with muted colors and tidier, narrower, often square-ended styles. Conservative leather ties also first saw the light of day.

The 1960s, 1970s, and 1980s

The 1960s and its flower power rebellion made ties, which represented traditional patriarchal authority and structure, somewhat unfashionable. The anti-tie movement gained speed in the 1970s.

What tie trends did exist in the 1960s, like many things, took their design cues from hippie counterculture. Ties were farcically wide, colors were vivid at best and often very gaudy, and print styles derived from nature—flowers and animals, bold geometrics—and a variety of ethnic textile patterns. The "kipper tie," which was up to a six inches wide, became and stayed popular through the late 1970s, when the leather tie—first seen in the 1950s but now reincarnated in a plethora of outlandish colors—also regained a grip it held on to into the 1980s. The 1980s, of course, ushered in a truly dreadful fashion period and led to some truly dreadful ties. One great thing happened for ties during this decade, though—Hermès launched its signature pattern of small repeated animal motifs, a style that remains elegant and whimsical, slightly offbeat but well within the bounds of convention.

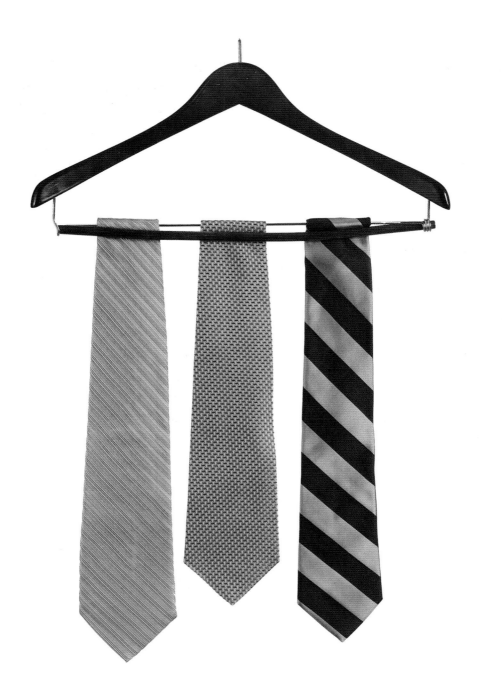

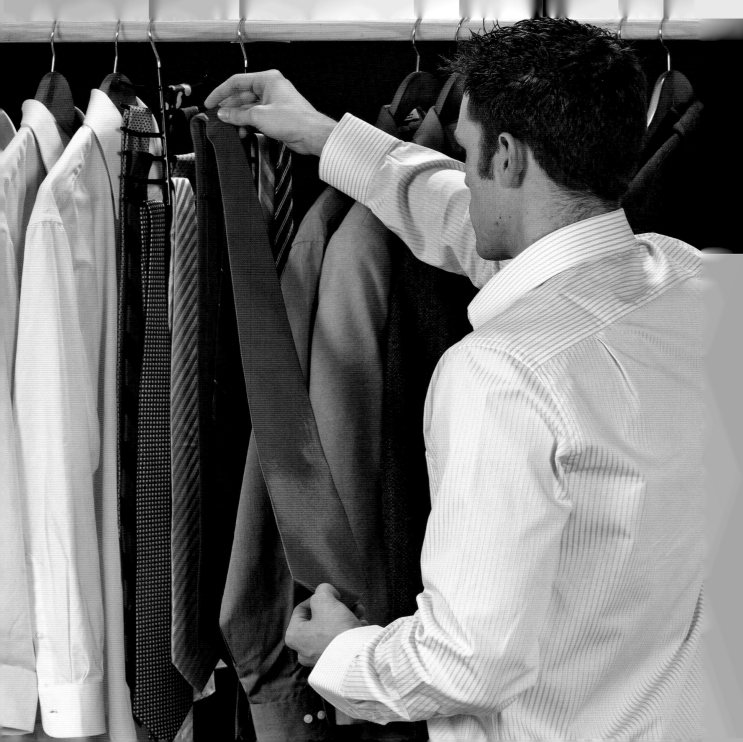

7.
how to **CARE** for ties

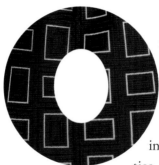

NCE YOU'VE PUT SOME TIME, ENERGY, AND money into creating a respectable tie wardrobe, you want the ties to last. As with all matters of apparel, the first step to ensuring that a tie has a long life is investing in one that is well made. Buying ties of high quality greatly increases the chances that they'll hold up better over a long period of regular wear—that is, stress to the tie's fabric that affects its shape, the intermittent cocktail or soup spill, and so on. But quality alone won't keep the tie looking good. No tie will last forever, and some will be rendered obsolete by virtue of pattern, color, or your own evolving tastes, but a properly cared-for tie will keep its texture and color longer and thus keep you looking good longer, too.

Handle your ties with kid gloves and they will wear well with age.

WEAR

Few men put much thought into what happens to a tie during the course of a day's wear, and good thing: The world, indeed, offers up far more weighty and tantalizing matters for contemplation. But a moment's reflection on the following items won't divert your attention for too long or too far from the finer points of culture and commerce. You'll just wind up looking better while you ponder them.

Never knot your silk tie too tightly. Though doing this might give you the feeling that the tie will stay knotted better during the day, in fact it won't. What it will do, if you do it repeatedly, is indelibly crease the tie's fabric, giving rise to tiny rips and tears. (Note: This doesn't apply to knitted silk ties, the slightly slippery texture of which requires a slightly tighter knot.)

At the end of the day, undo the tie properly and hang it up. Ease—don't yank—the tie ends gently out of their knot. This rule also applies to evenings' ends, regardless of the drinks tally. Only by hanging the tie will it regain its

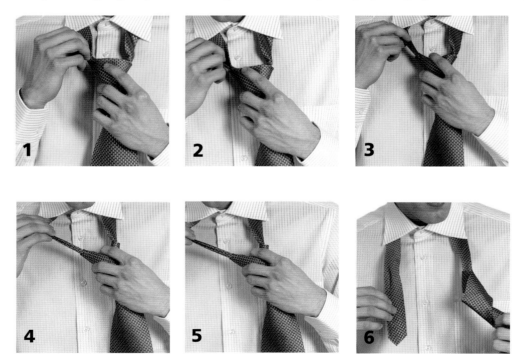

shape and its wrinkling be minimized, both immediately and over time.

Don't wear the same tie for two consecutive days. Apart from the looks askance you'll get at the office, this practice, if made routine, will eventually tire the tie out.

CLEANING AND PRESSING

How do you deal with a silk tie that's been sidelined by a food stain or seems rumpled beyond repair? Reports from the field indicate that there's no absolute consensus. One school of thought dictates sending the tie to the dry cleaner; another rules that no tie should ever be sent to the dry cleaner, from which it is sure to return ruined. As with most things, the reality is a little less cut-and-dried. Silk stains easily, and certain stains never seem to entirely disappear the way you'd like. But you needn't toss the tie out the minute it hosts a splotch of hors d'oeuvre from the office holiday party. Wrinkles are easier to get rid of. Below are some simple guidelines to help you keep your ties clean and wrinkle free.

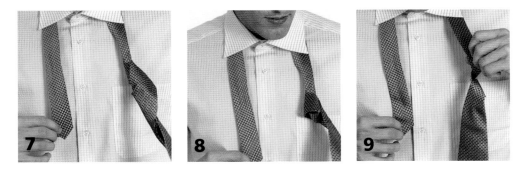

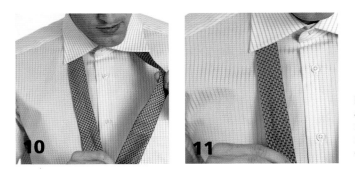

Remove a tie by first loosening it at the neck line, then pulling the narrow end through the knot, as this method prevents stretching of fabric and seams.

Ties don't go in the washing machine—not the one at home or at the professional laundry. Likewise, they mustn't be hand washed. These approaches may get the stain out, but they'll also result in a tie whose parts shrink disproportionately.

If you stain your tie with something greasy (such as steak fat or lipstick) or dark (such as red wine or ink), it's probably time to retire the tie. With this or a milder stain, you can try dabbing a tiny bit of water on the spot and very gently rubbing the tie's fabric against itself where the stain is, or using a slightly damp cloth to do the same. This valiant effort may or may not work; if it doesn't, you have a couple of options. Don't try to get the spot out with commercial stain remover or club soda. If you live in a major urban center, you can take the tie to a specialty dry cleaning service that deals with ties only. In New York, for example, Tiecrafters, a ties-only cleaning service, is the tie's best hope for resurrection. Otherwise, take the tie to the best dry cleaner you can find. Often, better dry cleaners will advertise that they "specialize" in ties. This may or may not actually be true, but you're better off with this approach than taking the tie to any old cleaner where, sadly, it may well come out looking as bad or worse than when it went in. Many men never have their ties cleaned. They simply wear them until the first signs of shabbiness or stain appear, and out they go.

Ironing your ties is generally a bad idea. One safe way to get creases out is to turn the steam on high and hold the iron just above the wrinkle in the tie. In a pinch, you can go heavy on the steam button and use an iron to dewrinkle your tie. Don't make this a regular practice, as (a) in the worst-case scenario you'll get a blackened tie and (b) it will wear the tie out more quickly. Also, be careful how you iron, because an absolutely flat tie won't hang naturally when you put it back on. There is actually such a thing as a tie press that you can buy for use at home—it works for ties made of silk and other materials and gets the tie looking smooth as new. But since the odds are high you may never invest in your very own tie press, here's an alternative method. If the tie is more wrinkled than an evening's hang will cure, try the following: Turn your shower on as hot as it can get; drape the tie over a hanger and hang it out of the water's reach, at the end of the shower opposite from the shower head; and leave it there for ten to twenty minutes. Remove the tie and lay it flat on a bureau or counter to dry, and you'll be good to go, without a wrinkle in sight.

STORAGE

In a just world, a man shouldn't have to worry about how his ties are stored. Nevertheless, you should pay a modicum of attention to the guidelines that follow. Read them once and they'll be second nature, and you'll spend less time buying new ties because the old ones will still be in good shape.

At home, ties are best stored in a closet. Keeping them in the dark slows the fabric's fading process. Circular swivel tie racks, which allow you to hang several ties lengthwise, are great, as the ties don't slip off of them, and they keep your ties all in one place. The next best bet is a regular old-fashioned hanger—drape the tie evenly over the metal frame so that it doesn't slip off and wind up crumpled on the floor. If for some reason you've got nowhere to hang ties, lay them flat in a drawer. Knitted ties should always be stored flat or carefully rolled in a drawer to prevent them from bagging and stretching disproportionately.

There are a couple of ways to handle tie storage when you're on the road. You can go the proper route and buy a special leather tie case or bag that allows the ties to lay flat, secured by horizontal straps. These will tuck easily into your suitcase and keep the ties in more or less immaculate condition. If that seems like too much effort, the old standby works perfectly well, too: Roll the ties in loose coils and pop them in your shoes, close enough together so they don't come unrolled, but not too squished (assuming, of course, that the shoes' insides aren't terribly malodorous). They should look good as new when you unpack them and get dressed for a business meeting or special occasion.

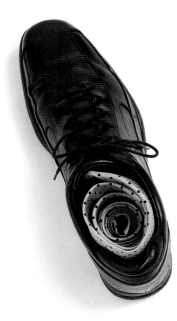

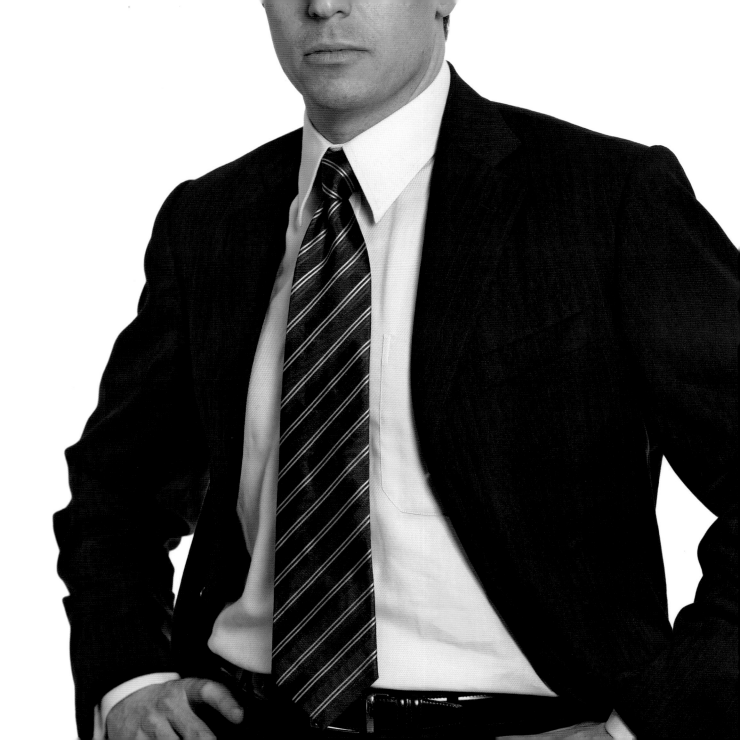

BIBLIOGRAPHY

The Book of Ties by Davide Mosconi and Riccardo Villarosa, Tie Rack Ltd., 1985

Chic Simple: Dress Smart Men by Kim Johnson Gross and Jeff Stone, Grand Central Publishing, 2002

Chic Simple: Men's Wardrobe by Kim Johnson Gross and Jeff Stone, Alfred A. Knopf, 2000

Chic Simple: Shirt and Tie by Michael Solomon, Alfred A. Knopf, 1993

Dressing the Man by Alan Flusser, HarperCollins, 2002

The 85 Ways to Tie a Tie by Thomas Fink and Yong Mao, Fourth Estate/HarperCollins, 2001

Esquire's Encyclopedia of 20th Century Men's Fashions by O. E. Schoeffler and William Gale, McGraw-Hill, 1973

Fashion for Men: An Illustrated History by Diana de Marly, Holmes and Meier, 1985

A History of Men's Fashion by Farid Chenoune, Flammarion, 1993

How to Tie Ties by Michael Adam, Sterling Publishing, 1996

The Indispensable Guide to Classic Men's Clothing by Josh Karlen and Christopher Sulavik, Tatra Press, 1999

The Little Book of Ties by Francois Chaille, Flammarion, 2001

Maximum Style by Perry Garfinkel, Brian Chichester, and the editors of Men's Health Books, Rodale Press, 1997

Style and the Man by Alan Flusser, Villard, 1988

The Style Guy by Glenn O'Brien, Ballantine, 2000

The Tie: Trends and Traditions by Sarah Gibbings, Barrons, 1990

Ties of Distinction by Christopher Sells, Schiffer Publishing, 1999

20th Century Neckties: Pre-1955 by Roseann Ettinger, Schiffer Publishing Ltd., 1998

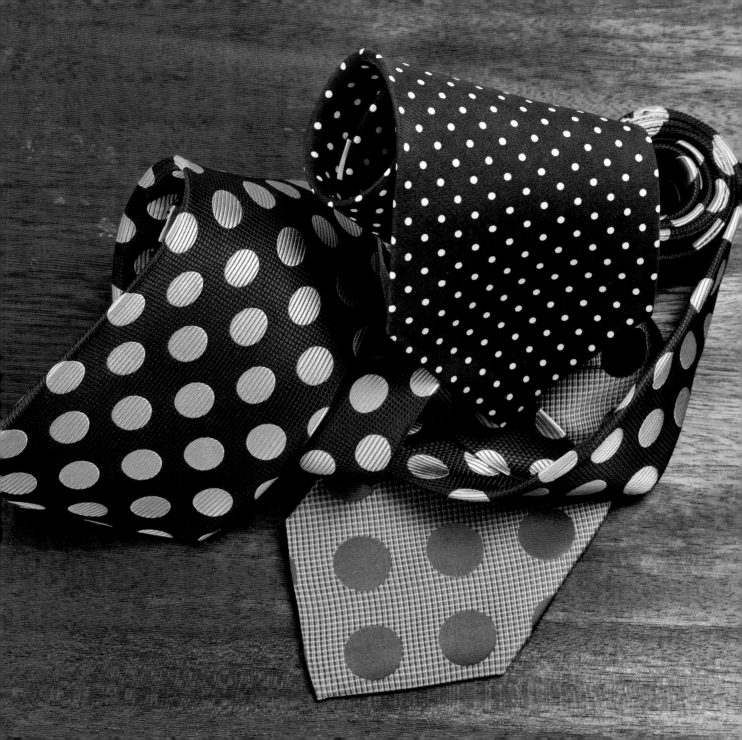

INDEX

INDEX